CW01184411

AS GOOD AS IT GETS

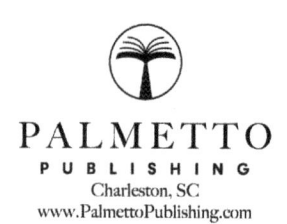

PALMETTO
PUBLISHING
Charleston, SC
www.PalmettoPublishing.com

Copyright © 2024 by Frank J. Brescia

All rights reserved.
This book or any portion thereof may not be reproduced or used in any manner whatsoever without the express written permission of the publisher except for the use of brief quotations in a book review.

Hardcover ISBN: 979-8-8229-4172-4
Paperback ISBN: 979-8-8229-4173-1
eBook ISBN: 979-8-8229-4174-8

AS GOOD AS IT GETS

The Evolving Thoughts of a Deathwatcher

FRANK J. BRESCIA,
MD, MA, FACP

For Christie

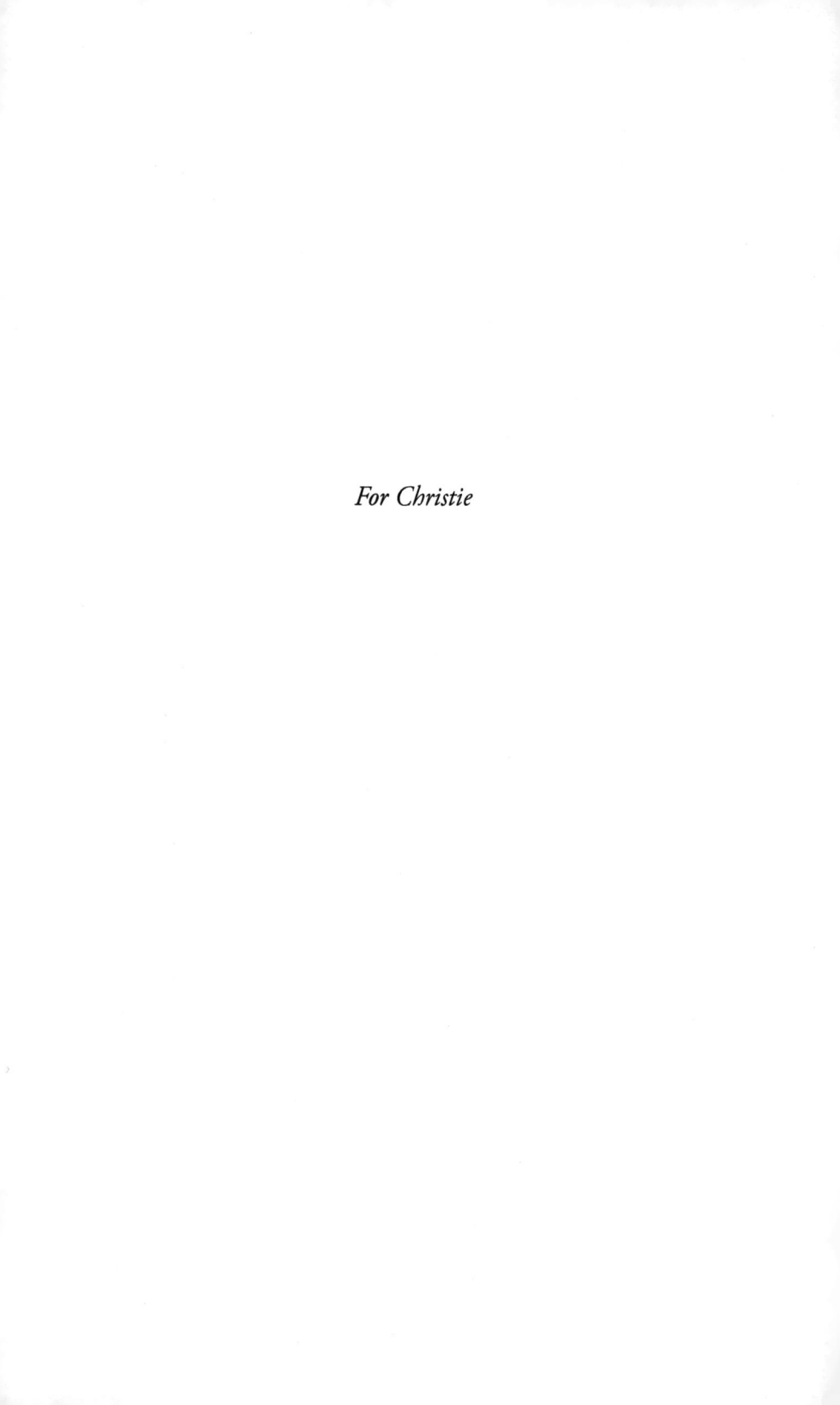

CONTENTS

PREFACE	1
INTRODUCTION	7
PART I: *Thoughts About Me*	11
PART II: *Becoming a Doctor*	38
PART III: *Learning about Caring for the Dying*	46
PART IV: *Vietnam*	56
PART V: *Jane — Reflections on Love and Loss, Grief, and Guilt*	82
PART VI: *Postdeath Reflections*	113
PART VII: *Principles for Dying*	127
PART VIII: *Suffering: A Test of Character*	143
PART IX: *Random Reflections — Trying to Pull It Together*	153
PART X: *New Life: It Begins Again*	165
PART XI: *What's Next?*	177
FURTHER READINGS	181
ABOUT THE AUTHOR	185
ACKNOWLEDGEMENTS	186

PREFACE

It was only after my wife, Jane's death from breast cancer in late June 2013, when I was truly alone, with the house empty of all kids and leftover mourners, that I began to reflect on my life with Jane, my terrible loss, my work as a cancer doctor, and finally my life as a whole. I wondered, What the hell just happened here? Everything seemed too weighty to matter any longer, and nothing seemed to make sense going forward. There was no road map. Call it confusion. Grief, loss, guilt, love, and a lack of purpose became the themes of my new solitude. And I got stuck in all remembrances of the past, the lost good moments, without any motivation to see a new day dawn. Even more, there was no hope for tomorrow, that tomorrow would be a better day than today. I had the luxury of time to do the business at hand—the undertaking, the memorial services, the disposing of worn and unworn clothing, and the addressing of the necessary paperwork of death. We had recently sold all our properties, and I was renting a large old home in downtown Charleston, South Carolina, that was just right for me and my two dogs, Max and Charlie. I had no one to offer advice to me or warnings or sympathies or anything. I was not eating too much. I was not eating too little. In some ways, it was the easiest of times. I was alone. Solitude brings on introspection and self-discovery. I had at least found that. I could walk the house freely in my underwear. What is better than that?

Coming from a large extended family, I'd seen people age, and I'd watched people die. Grandparents died first, then parents and friends. I witnessed firsthand the casualties of the war in Vietnam. I treated patients who died. But nothing was like the loss of my wife, Jane. Maybe it was because she died from breast cancer, the disease I was supposed to know most about—a cruel gesture of the universe. Why was her death so much more difficult to bear? Perhaps it was the protracted time of watching her slip away, feeling the loss of her laughter. I saw nothing redemptive in her pain and battle. And though I wasn't angry at a God I hadn't prayed to in a long time, I questioned the apathy and indifference of a divine presence. I was upset that there was no God that could help right the wrong, or worse, that there was a God that was blind and deaf to any pleas for help. Why was she here only to be taken away? After all, who the hell was I to expect prayers to be listened to, or even better, answered?

As humans, we rehearse all the loss experienced in a lifetime—in my case, all those I loved, and especially now, Jane. "Why?" was the question. Had I added value and meaning to her life, or to the life of anyone I had known, for that matter? What does this reality soup we live in mean? I realized I was not smart enough to figure this one out, but was it so absurd to ask questions?

I was looking for an explanation for everything! How absurd! I was seeking a narrative of our cosmic history and the evolution of conscious awareness, and that awareness looked back, trying to understand it all through scientific thought, religious beliefs, and philosophical explanations. And of course, there was the matter of understanding the mystery of just being. Not too shabby a quest!

I began to recall not only my life with Jane but also all those who had mattered to me over my lifetime—who had taught me the "how" of being. I realized how many mentors, teachers, and role models we have over a timeline of living.

Even our children refresh the course about love, sacrifice, devotion, and fidelity and perhaps enhance meaning. The interconnectedness of all of us is crucial, giving value to each of us. And I thought about love. Even if the universe seemed loveless, cold, unmoved, and seemingly uncaring about me, I seemed to care. I thought that was a good thing. I was well aware of the truth and reality of what love is, as sure as I knew the majesty of smelling coffee in the morning. The physical death of someone loved never removes the reality of that person's presence and existence.

I was always interested in the big questions. I had decided to get a master's degree in philosophy at Fordham University years after becoming a medical oncologist. I faced the day-to-day problems of our human frailty, and I was seeking meaning. Study gave me the opportunity to have someone smarter than I explain the philosophical explanations I was reading. My patients filled in the gaps of the human condition. I had seen the futility of war in Vietnam during my twenties, and it forced upon me an experience not many have seen or need to see. And through it all, I have witnessed death and dying in various forms, which have always, always left me seeking answers to the query of what's next for us. Will the stuff that makes me who I am go beyond the grave? Will I dream? Will I keep some form of awareness and my conscious self? And more importantly, will my Easter-people religion—my inherited Catholic faith, which believes in the resurrection of the dead—allow me to experience again those I so loved in life? Will all of us, only then, find purpose in this existence we share? Wouldn't that be nice?

In 2020, I was asked to speak at an international conference in Sapporo, Japan. The meeting was intended to explore spirituality in medicine, a subject that has recently been recognized as important by academic medical centers such as Duke University School of Medicine and Harvard Medical School. My topic was the "Intersection of Medicine, Philosophy, and Religion." The meeting unfortunately had to be cancelled due to the COVID pandemic, but I was already trying to formulate ideas around this subject. I began to think seriously about my own take on things as a medical oncologist. Did I have something rich to contribute, and could I say it better than it was said before? That seemed the harder challenge.

I began to think of the work I have done, how it has changed over the last fifty years, and more importantly, how it has changed and challenged me. I've come to believe that time is an illusion and all the moments one lives really happen all at once. My past is as real as my present. The nows of our days are all now. I believe this is what Einstein's theory of relativity showed. After all, someone on a faraway galaxy looking at Earth is seeing my past or the dinosaurs' past as now. My reflection began as an evolution of the thoughts of a death watcher. After all, the child I was is still part of my reflective self. I acknowledge from the start that my narrative may be strabismic and bumfuzzled (two of my favorite words) but hopefully also explanatory and agreeable. As I have ripened, I have become able to see my life, if not more clearly, at least with more nuance. It is always now.

My professional life now consists of caring for patients with breast cancer, with either early or late disease. Some have been cured. Some have died. Sometimes they have died old, and too often they have succumbed too soon, leaving behind too many of their now moments and unrealized memories. The stories of ordinary lives end too soon, and their epic books are forever closed. As a physician, I see patients in the most awful times of their lives, filled with pain, uncertainty, fear, confusion, anxiety, and hopelessness And yes, one of the profound, complicated duties of my profession is to instill back hope that, indeed, tomorrow will be better than today, or at least no worse. Threading the needle of hope can be difficult, especially when we know that hope can be the flip side of despair. We can wish for something that we know is truly not possible. Sometimes, all that is wished for is for a tomorrow—whether that tomorrow is good or bad.

I recently walked through the connection between the university hospital and the cancer center where I work. On the second floor on the left as one enters the hospital is the morgue—the place where dead bodies are kept. A new large sign had been hung in the middle of the hallway: "Decedent Affairs." I passed the sign for several days, and I became irritated. What affairs do dead people have? What is wrong with the word "morgue"? I know what "morgue" means. I don't know what "decedent affairs" means. Do the dead have an interest in their affairs? Nothing spiritual here, I thought. This is a real frailty in our language. But what do I know, and why should I care? Because, I thought, it matters.

This is a story about me—not a heroic epic, but a narrative connected to the themes of my life around the problem of facing serious illness and the difficult journey of dying. It is a self-reflective narrative about life, loss, and grief—or at least my personal grief. Hopefully, it is a story about the search for the meaning of doctoring and caring for the seriously ill. It is also about the dreams and regrets of our lives—things we would like to do over. Can I offer wisdom?

I am blessed in being a physician, caring for people in the most difficult of times in their lives. Being a physician is a noble, almost spiritual endeavor in which my door should never be locked. Society has bestowed on me the privilege to know, dissect, and celebrate the most intimate of details in human stories. It has allowed me the incredible gift of touching others, as Adam would have touched the first man and woman for the first time. It is a honorable trade born out of hours of lost sleep, sacrificed relationships, and multiple twinklings of self-doubt. I have delivered new life into our world and given testimony of a life's last breath. In it all, I have seen the mystery of the cosmic balance sheet of gain and loss.

There are multiple rewards for being a physician. Society praises us for our skills, sacrifices, and relevance. I must confess that there is, especially realized over time, a real, sincere, powerful sense of satisfaction—a sense that in truly relieving pain and suffering in the darkest of times for people, you are, as a physician, made more whole. The time given away for study when you were younger has been more than amply rewarded in a life that is worth living. And isn't that enough and as good as it gets? Animals, we are told by the wisdom of Abraham Joshua Heschel, need to be satisfied. But we, as the most noble of beings, need to be needed. Yet most of us want independence and refuse to accept the help that may be required.

I began to scribble down notes about what I observed and about what I remembered as important in my life. What is it to have a life of worth? What is it to be a good physician, and more importantly, a good person? This, then, became a reflection, an evolution of the thoughts of a death watcher that grew out of my personal story as a physician, father, and husband. Could I make some sense of my time here, my losses, and my work to at least please myself? I knew from the outset I could not and would not find all the answers, but isn't it, I thought, better to at least ask the questions? These are those evolving, random thoughts of a death watcher. This is the product of my scribbled notes.

INTRODUCTION

I begin this meditation as an inward probing of what I have considered important in my life, with an attempt to understand my long journey of learning and witnessing life as a physician. Philosopher Robert Nozick starts his wonderful meditations in *The Examined Life* with "I want to think about living and what is important in life, to clarify my thinking and also my life." My personal reflection is a troubled clinician's deliberation with himself, born out of a need to better understand the nature of this work I do and my life. I have come to realize how closely my life and work are interwoven and connected. A life is a mosaic, much more a painting and portrait in progress and less a series of isolated photographs.

For over fifty years, I have been both a death watcher and a doctor watcher—approaching the human drama at the bedside of sick, hurting, and often dying patients, bringing my unique take on things, with lifelong collections of doubts, questions, prejudices, fears, memories, and unresolved issues about my own vulnerability. In my line of work, it has been difficult to avoid thinking about the things all of us want to avoid thinking about. Simply stated—what is it all about?

What does it all mean, and where do I fit in? Where are we ultimately going?

The premise of my examination is that if I, the physician, remain open to honest self-reflection—to the constant calls of my patients in distress—it will create an opportunity for me to become, not only a better physician, but a better person as well, because ultimately both the individual as a patient in need and I will face the same existential anxiety.

Jean-Paul Sartre echoed what we know—we have this human curse; we are condemned by the knowledge that someday we will cease to be. Just contemplate that certainty of fact. We have only to read the daily newspaper each morning. How can that be? Believe me—it is! In the 1970s, Ted Rosenthal, a young poet, who was dying of acute leukemia, asked, "How can I not be among you?" This one unimaginable, inevitable fact is always present, facing each and every one of us, our very futures. We have nothing our imaginations can prepare us with to help us envision what follows or compare it to any experience we've had—an unavoidable given. We must rejoice now for the joy of our next breath and not delay.

Writer Julian Barnes asks this question in his terrific book *Nothing To Be Frightened Of* "What is it about death that terrifies us?" Some of us fear an afterlife of eternal punishment and suffering, and others have an even more disturbing belief in a perpetual void—true nothingness. We become part of the earth and dirt, and we believe in the total loss of everything, with no interest or need for interest in anything—that is real loss. Some philosophers are materialists and dismiss any certitude of evidence for an immortal soul. I am not sure, but perhaps consciousness of some kind will continue, maybe because it has always been there as a universal and fundamental fact of the cosmos, here from the very beginning of time. Maybe that fact will give us continued existence in some form of afterlife. And then there is God, who, to many, will give us everlasting life because that is, they say, ultimately the reason we were created—to be with God.

We are told that to be a philosopher is to learn how to die. This is easier said than done and is certainly not something we can spend too much time dwelling upon, or else we would get little accomplished. One could rightly ask, "What's the point?" Perhaps it is not death so much that people fear, but rather the indignity of aging, sickness, and the process of dying, along with the realization that this is as good as it gets—the incompleteness of our lives, of what we should and could have done with our lives. How quickly does a life pass, with so much left to say and do. Death is not just a catastrophic biological event with such significance and permanence, but its gravity is also magnified by our inability to gather any of its meaning. As the New Testament explains, we ultimately must turn to seed and die before fruit can be borne, and therefore, the secret of the survival of the universe is for all of us to die and become fuel for our replacements. This is not a comforting thought, but I suspect it to be true. In the end, maybe it is our consciousness, self-awareness, and questioning about our existence that make the universe approve that we were here. Perhaps the cosmic mystery requires me to be aware, to know of its presence by giving me consciousness to see the beauty and order of the universe.

I have now reached an age where if I die, no one will likely suggest I went too soon. More likely, people may be surprised that I am still alive, which might be more disturbing. My qualifications to deal with these ultimate deep questions regarding life's meaning, death, God, and the cosmos are no better than anyone else's. I have no more expertise or wisdom than the next person. I'm certainly no deeper or intellectually or spiritually more sophisticated than the average—indeed, probably less so. I am a physician. I have treated sickness and pain, and I have seen the end of life. I have seen suffering in the Vietnam War and have feared dying in a foreign place. I have six children: four biological, one adopted, and one raised as my own since infancy. I have had a marriage annulled, I have had a divorce, and I have become a widower after twenty years of a terrific marriage. Even now, I am blessed with love and romance when I thought it was all gone. The potential to feel and experience love is unending.

Come take this journey with me. I have lived a reasonably long and interesting life as a physician, treating people with cancer and end-of-life issues. I am looked upon as a father and husband. I am not rich or famous, nor have I ever expected to be. I am loved deeply again by my wife Christie, and by my four daughters and two sons. I am, by temperament, a New Yorker, and by ethnicity, for better or worse, a product of genes from southern Italy. I love my Italian culture and food. I enjoy traveling, and I play the piano well enough for people to think that I'm good. I fake well. Despite this, I have tried to never fake life, family, work, or my close relationships with those I love. I have tried really hard to believe and look for the proofs that there is a God, but I still have doubts. Above all, I tend to think too much.

PART I:
Thoughts About Me

I was born two months after the Japanese attack on Pearl Harbor. My birth was a welcome event for two reasons. First, my parents were married on June 1, 1941, and I arrived on February 24, 1942—you do the math. Second, more importantly, I was a reason to keep my father out of the war, at least until 1944.

Fables surrounding my conception were family lore. I was told my father was with his father's youngest brother, Uncle Tony, a mere few hours before I came to be. He and Aunt Philomena had no children, and Uncle Tony was speaking with his newly married nephew and stressing the importance of having children—do it right away. My father, always ready for the dramatics, came home to the house owned by my mother's parents and announced with an apparent shout of confidence, "This is the night!" I know no more.

Many years later, after my father died, I invited my mom to a somewhat formal welcoming cocktail party in the late afternoon to celebrate my new position at a hospital in Atlanta. My wife, Jane, joined me as well. Somewhere in the middle portion of this quiet event with all my new physician and administrative coworkers, I noted to my wife that my mother was missing. She was not gone but appeared to be holding court at the other end of the room, the center of attention, surrounded by these new colleagues. My wife entered this circle and came back out smiling—my mom was talking about my "conception history." I never asked what actually was presented that nice afternoon. But apparently, it was enough to draw an audience.

I come from European peasant stock; both sides of my heritage were from the same poor farming country of southern Italy—a region called Basilicata and a small town called Aliano, southeast of Rome. This certainly was one of the poorest areas of Italy and drove the Italian migration to the United States in the early part of the last century. My mother's mother, Rose, arrived in New York as a child of four in 1904. Her husband, my maternal grandfather, Giuseppe Colucci, came later, although I was told that his father had come and gone, making and losing a fortune in the New World. There was always a hint of stories regarding womanizing, although I'm not sure if this is true. My great-grandfather, Joseph Brescia, was born in the 1860s, married an orphan, Anna, and came to New York to start a delivery-carting business. Brescia is the name of a large northern Italian city in the more industrialized and cultural center of Italy. How the name came to my family is unknown to me. It is typically a Jewish-Italian name—often the case if the name is of a specific place. I'm told that Joseph was Jewish and his brothers settled in Argentina. My great-grandfather had a tragic end. As the story goes, he came home from work on a hot July day. Anna was cooking supper, and my great-grandfather, tired, went out on the fire escape to take a nap and stay cool. He was summoned to come inside once dinner was ready; then he became disoriented, still groggy from the nap and perhaps a glass of wine, fell off the fire escape, and was impaled by the spiked metal fence below—in full view of his son, Frank, who was playing out front. There was talk regarding sending the children, Frank, Anthony, Louis, and Mamie, to Argentina, as there was no great social net to help my great-grandmother survive. I was told they did not want the kids brought up in Argentina as Jews. She washed clothes for pay and survived.

My father, Freddie or Alfredo (like in *The Godfather*), never made it to high school. He had multiple talents in the trades, played multiple musical instruments, and had a reasonably successful house-painting job when I was born. He was also a self-taught artist. My mother's brother Louis was a master carpenter and built homes in the Bronx and probably also kept my father's house-painting business afloat. My mother worked all her life as a dressmaker, working in the 1940s sweatshops that they write about, making pennies per dress. I remember as a kid visiting the "factory"—hot and noisy, with unending tables of women sewing on these deafening sewing machines. I realized later in life why the television was so damn loud! She was a good dressmaker, and my pants always had impeccable cuffs—and my children, new dresses. I can echo similar themes about my mom as those Woody Allen used to describe his mother—God, carpeting, cleanliness, and above all, order, everything in its rightful place. I had the neatest, cleanest bedroom of all my friends, and if I, God forbid, had gone blind, I could have found everything in its place—even my underwear, folded neatly right where it should be. My father often complained that if he dared to go use the bathroom at night, he would return to find the bed made.

I survived my childhood in the northeast Bronx, growing up happily nurtured by the tribal conditions afforded me. The B trolley's last stop was at our street, East 229th Street, and the White Plains elevated IRT train and Third Avenue line ended at 241st Street. A kid could go anywhere and everywhere on fun transportation.

My parents rented a small two-bedroom apartment on the first floor of my mother's parents' home—813 East 229th Street. Our household included my grandparents in the basement, where all the real living took place; it had the kitchen and the dining/living room, separated by a door leading to the unfinished basement area. Here, coal would be delivered by a chute, and my grandfather Giuseppe each year would make two barrels of wonderful dry red wine. The small backyard had a grapevine awning, and behind that small space was an impressive vegetable garden on one side and a parklike flower garden on the other. This was my world. The other relatives living in this three-story brick building included my maternal uncles, Louis and Joe, my maternal aunts, Millie and Diana, and my four cousins. The hallway steps were marble, and my grandfather every Saturday morning thoroughly mopped them in his dress pants and white dress shirt. In the identical twin brick building to the left, twenty feet away, lived my maternal great-grandparents, my maternal grandmother's two brothers, their wives, and their children. Five more cousins were added here. Childhood diseases came to us kids as expected, without any fanfare or concern. Doctors were seen only if you were bleeding to a near-transfusion level. No one fussed if you had fever, vomiting, rashes, swollen anything, or much of anything. I don't recall my parents having regular checkups. It was easy living.

We were the first in the neighborhood to have a television—probably around 1948. It was an RCA ten-inch screen with initially one station, NBC. Most of us listened to the radio—*The Lone Ranger, The Shadow, Suspense, Inner Sanctum*. My mother was addicted to the soaps of the day. I remember late afternoons watching *The Howdy Doody Show*. This program first aired in December 1947—I had to have been on five or six years old. There was also the unthinkable idea of watching Arturo Toscanini leading the NBC Symphony Orchestra in the late afternoon. A puppet show and Beethoven all in one afternoon! There was this one station to watch on a ten-inch screen—what wonders would there be?

Music, like food, was built into daily life. Musical sound was always in our house. My grandparents and my aunts and uncles—all of whom lived within blocks of one another—always had the radio on, listening to opera on Saturdays sponsored by Texaco. There were *Make Believe Ballroom*, baritones, and a young Tony Bennett. Later there were new rock and roll sounds like "Earth Angel." But always Sinatra! My father brought home a used upright rebuilt piano before I started school, and I began my piano lessons with Mrs. Kunua across our block on 229th Street. I played "Indian Dance Song" at The Town Hall on 43rd Street in Manhattan on a Sunday summer afternoon at my first recital. I couldn't reach the foot pedal in my clean, white, short pants, but I was good and made no mistakes. My father even came, which in itself was a surprise.

I later—near nine or ten years of age—took lessons with Professor Franco in the Bronx. My parents must have seen something in me. I would take my music books and walk alone along White Plains Road from 229th Street downtown to 217th Street to his private house on the second floor. I made it to Czerny exercises—these were practical piano exercises by composer Carl Czerny, who lived in the early 1800s. They usually begin with Opus 599, which introduces the student to the technical aspects of the piano. Things did not go well with Professor Franco and me, and only recently did I forgive myself for not being that good—missing notes or timing—because I believe I was nearsighted. I needed glasses. How is that for an excuse? Often, my lesson was interrupted by my being sent to his large screened-in porch room filled with many singing birds in cages, where I would need to write the musical notes down on paper. This was not going well—humiliation, even for a ten-year-old. I still have a photograph he took of me playing the piano—I always felt, correctly or not, that he wanted to document his worst pupil. On his grand black piano where I took my lessons was a black-and-white photograph of Professor Franco's daughter playing the piano. She looked serious, and though he never spoke about her, I always assumed she was much better than I was.

My final piano teacher did not last long because my piano caught on fire and was totaled. How, you ask? There I was, in our cold basement, on a winter day, practicing my lessons. My teacher was due soon. We had an electric space heater that kept me comfortable. It's hard playing with a coat. However, I didn't recognize how warm the upper keys were getting, as I didn't need to play them. There was this sudden loud whoosh and flash and flames and heat! I leaped away. My mother, home upstairs, was down quickly. The curtains on the windows now also were ablaze. The flames quickly went out with not much water. The smell of ash was obvious. My mother did not yell at me—she was too happy that I was all right and the house had not burned to the ground. I had not a mark on my body. My piano teacher was out of a job with me. I would have to deal with my father later because he was convinced I had done this deliberately. My piano was gone. That would be my last formal lesson.

    I do remember my parents bringing home an accordion. They obviously felt I needed some discipline to keep me out of trouble. There was no way I was going to play an accordion. Yes, it has a keyboard like a piano, but the keys release air through reeds inside, just like a woodwind instrument. I agreed to take lessons if they also got me a monkey! My formal lesson days were over.

    I was not a tough kid growing up in the Bronx. I had my fair share of bullying, but it was never anything lasting or too terrible to handle. The family members that I knew were gentle people and not prone to initiate fights with anyone in the neighborhood. My father was the most volatile of his five brothers and my mother's two brothers. He had a menacing appearance somewhat like Tony Soprano's but a personality more like Oliver Hardy's. However, as kids, my cousins and I did not want to be on his wrong side. There was a good-natured, gentle side of him, but always a potential smoldering explosion ready to erupt, if provoked. He instilled awe in me with his presence, and he got the respect he demanded. There was often laughter surrounding his presence and always surprise at his entry into a room. Was he the model dad you see on television? No. He had little patience with me or, I suspect, even with my brother. He was not the model dad to teach me to catch a ball, ride a bike, swim, or drive a car. He never took me to a ball game, fishing, boating, hunting, or even to a movie, to church, or to any school event I can remember. We would visit family, and the family was huge! He was the storyteller of the family lore.

My father was not an ethical model dad either, I may add. I remember once going with him to a large hardware store in Mount Vernon, New York. I was maybe nine or ten years old. He and my uncles were very much interested in setting up Lionel trains at Christmastime, and they usually would start the layout in my grandparents' home in late October. This hardware store was having a 50 percent off sale on Lionel trains, with the markdowns written on the boxes. When we came to the Lionel train section, the boxes had the half-price markdown noted. For example, a train engine was selling for forty dollars that had formerly cost eighty dollars. My father took a marker and wrote "$20" and placed a cross on the markdown that said "$40." He whispered for me to say nothing as we checked out, paying twenty dollars for the eighty-dollar train engine. He never told my mother. I never told my mother. I knew it was wrong. Was this the lesson I was taught? I had a new train!

My father grew up in the tenement housing of East Harlem at 110th Street. He swam in the East River like many of the boys of the day. Comedian George Carlin talked about how they increased their immune potential by swimming in sewage. I remember my dad telling me that he and his friend went out, at his friend's request, to find this guy to murder. Who knows why? My father's friend was intent on killing him for a reason I can't remember or was never told. My father told me that, thank God, they never did find him, or he probably would have been still in jail. This friend apparently did eventually kill someone and was locked up at the time I was a kid. I never saw any more evil in my dad than changing a train box price.

When I was picked on by kids bigger than I was, it was upsetting, and as a kid I kept quiet. There was this one broad, fat, strong neighborhood kid named Auggie. He was unrelenting to us younger kids with name calling and shoving. My father saw it one day and took me aside: "He is never going to stop unless you tell him to stop, and if you need to fight him, you fight him!" My father suggested a two-by-four piece of wood could help. I wasn't ready for that. However, the next time Auggie came down on me, I shoved and attacked back. Although I got the worst of the fight, I succeeded in giving him a few good punches to the face and giving him a bloody nose. He never bothered me again. My father, from the window of our house, watched me lose this fight, but I won the war of boyhood bullying. I never used the two-by-four piece of wood. Auggie and I became friends. *And the lion and the lamb will sleep together.*

We did get another rebuilt, secondhand piano. My dad played reasonably well by ear, but he was all self-taught. Unlike me, he also played the guitar, harmonica, and drums. It was good to have the piano back in the house because now I could play without the pressure of books and lessons and metronomes and giving up an hour and having to show off what I'd recently learned to any visitor. But I did play, and like my father, I became self-taught to fake well. Every time I ran into a real musician, I would watch and ask questions regarding chord changes and what to do with my left hand. I would buy sheet music to help me set new challenges for myself. Finally, in high school, the piano helped me to engage with others I otherwise would have never bothered to know. It also allowed me to be quiet at parties; I didn't need to talk—I could just play alone in the corner whatever I wanted to play. And I always said, "I'm really not that good—no lessons. I'm faking," which was all very true.

But the truth was, my faking was getting better. Finally, by my junior year of high school, I was invited to join a singing group for a high school entertainment show at the end of the school year, and the Fascinations was born. We made three demonstration records with some songs I had cowritten—usual rock and roll stuff of the fifties. We were not that bad, and my father was becoming concerned that I was abandoning my dream of going to college and my goal of becoming a physician. We were good, but not *that* good. That dream of stardom was never to take real form. It took me out of my comfortable shell of only books and study. I had become a good student by this time. I was quite content to leave my limited musical career and move on. My high school friends all scattered, and death had come to the Fascinations. My father was relieved.

My piano has always been there for me. I'm not sure if people who don't play an instrument can understand this connection. I thank my mother for taking the time to make me practice when I first started. It would require an hour—"One hour," she would say—each day. And with the metronome keeping a consistent tempo, I would not go too slow or too fast. I hear it now as I write, as the pendulum of my clock goes tick-tock. Kelsey Grammer said, "Prayer is when you talk to God. Meditation is when you're listening. Playing the piano allows you to do both at the same time."

I remember many years later, when I was in Vietnam, missing the feel and sound of the piano—this withdrawal longing of being unable to touch the keys and hear the feedback resonance of the notes and chords. I had been there almost ten months. Now stationed safely in Cam Ranh Bay, I would walk or even hitchhike to the next village. Not far from our base, I found a small, locked, closed white chapel on the road. Looking in the window, I could see the piano in the front of the building near the small altar. It was as if heroin were calling my name. Alone, I was able to open a window, climb over a small cabinet, and get inside. No alarms! No one around. I was able to play unbothered. An audience of me. I can't recall what I played, but I stayed nearly an hour the first visit. It was time to leave before I was discovered, to go back out the window, but I would return many times until my addiction was healed and I would go home. It was an old piano, certainly out of tune, but it sounded wonderful to my deluded ear. I loved that little chapel and thanked it for making me whole again.

All the notes in music pages are absolutely laid out for you. There should be little "free choice" in playing the piece as written by the composer. It is written in such a way for a reason. The notes and timing are there for you to play. In life, too, the notes and rhythm of our days are laid out for us. It is a matter of our unique individual techniques and interpretations to make the difference. That's how we can tell who is really good. Music gave this kid confidence that he could do other things.

My parents seemed happy and content. I never had any fear or threat that their marriage wouldn't last. On the contrary, they often would ask each other if they would remarry if the other one died. I always found the questioning strange. The answer was always a resounding no, and I believe that they were answering honestly. They had apparently met at a family wedding in 1940 where both were in the wedding party. They obviously knew of each other, as their families were tied to the same town, Aliano, in the old country. They spoke the same dialect, and their mothers made the Sunday "gravy" (i.e., the meat tomato sauce) the same way. There was palpable attraction toward each other, yet they were very different—my mother reserved, neat, patient, religious, and quiet, and my father not. He would start fights with the New Jersey toll collectors about giving them the twenty-five cents if the traffic line was too long. In his house-painting business, if a customer wished him to paint a room a certain color that my father thought not quite right, he wouldn't paint! My parents had their disagreements—most often my father's fault. An example of a disagreement: they were having an early dinner—they always ate at an ungodly early hour. My father was reading the monthly *Reader's Digest*, where the cover showed a beautiful winter snow scene displaying colorful pheasants scattered about the drawing. My father asked if my mother liked the picture, and apparently, she said yes. Wrong answer. Dinner was over, and my mom was headed to the grocery store to shop. I don't know how long she was out shopping, but let's give it two to two and a half hours. On her arrival back home, she was greeted by a new living-room and front-entrance mural of a beautiful snow scene and large (very large) pheasants scattered about the room. I don't believe they spoke for a couple of weeks, but the pheasants stayed over a year.

I was an only child until my brother was born in September 1957. I was entering medical school when my brother, Ronnie, started kindergarten. One week before my father died unexpectedly, he sat across from me talking about his life. This was August 1977. My third child, Michaelann, had just been born and was still not home from the hospital. My father talked openly that Saturday—quite unlike him—about my mother and about children. He was happy I was having a larger family and said that he would have wanted more kids. My mother could not imagine the chaos and mess that more kids would bring. My father was happy my brother was here—I was a necessity, but my brother contingent! He became a much softer dad and certainly more engaging. He would be dead before my brother was twenty. My oldest daughter, Andria, is my only child who has fleeting memories of my dad. She was four when he died.

The old among us—aunts, uncles, and widows in the family living among the tribe—would die and be laid to rest in the living room for their wakes. Nothing seemed different about them—the dead person, previously alive, was in the corner of the room not saying very much. We slept upstairs—the dead rested downstairs.

I'm a proud product of the New York City public education system—P.S. (Public School) 21. The school was between my two sets of grandparents' homes—225th Street close to White Plains Road, where the Wakefield elevated IRT line and station still are today. My father's parents lived on 224th Street, one block south. The school had a great large playground with all a kid needed to hurt himself – fantastic monkey bars! In the late spring, they would have a huge water sprinkler to cool us down. This was primarily an Italian American neighborhood—not as Italian as Arthur Avenue in the Bronx, but close. For the longest time, I thought everyone's name ended in a vowel. There wasn't a great variation in first names—Mario, Anthony, Vinnie, Auggie, Frankie, Louie—or in nicknames, which were usually given for some anatomical defect—Lefty, Tiny, Limpy, Shorty, Curly, Red. One could hear Italian spoken as one walked to school, passing homes with fenced-off lots of growing vegetables. These fields were replaced in the late fifties with the construction of multiple attached homes. The Bronx quickly lost its rural-like feel.

I was neither encouraged nor discouraged from learning Italian. My grandparents spoke it to each other, but rarely to me—unless I had done something wrong. My parents spoke Italian, but only to the elders. The war may have created this need to spare the language and—wanting to become part of the melting pot—speak English. I suspect their Italian—since they had lived in the country four decades by the time I came along—was tainted and bastardized. I do regret not learning such a beautiful language. I always missed not being able to explain something in two different languages. I would tell Jane that everything said in Italian sounds lyrical, filled with romance, and everything said in her German sounds like "Where are your papers?"

I admit I was an awful student in grammar school—undisciplined with really no motivation. I had concluded I wasn't good at anything. Perhaps a civil service position was my future—drive the subway and become a motorman. My grandfather, Frank, worked for the IRT and would take me as a small kid to the subway work yards. What fun running through empty subway cars! I don't remember being pressured to do homework—especially in contrast to my cousins, who were all attending neighborhood Catholic schools. I don't know what my parents were expecting of me—it never was a topic of family discussion, at least during my early years. I don't think that they didn't care—they had no reference about my educational needs and goals. My mother worked and came home late, made dinner, cleaned, and went to bed to face another day. In the morning my father would leave me with my maternal grandmother, who would overindulge me at breakfast and lunchtime. I remember having espresso for breakfast, sometimes with a raw egg tossed in—a good diuretic load for a little kid. I had to pee as soon as I got to school! I was ready to face the world.

My mother seemed much more interested in the immediacy of my cleanliness, hygiene, and appearance than in my far-off future. I remember when my father brought home a set of the *Encyclopedia Britannica* and the *Book of Knowledge*—which, somehow, I was to start absorbing. They never did read to me—not that I'm complaining; it's just a fact. I'm not sure any of my cousins were ever read to either. It was a different time.

A word about the movies. When I was really young, the radio was the window of the world or the theater of the mind. Television was yet to be born, and movies were very special. In New York, the Manhattan theaters would show one new movie, and it would stay for weeks, depending on the popularity of that film. This was something special, like going to the theater to see a play. Some theaters, like the Paramount, would often have a show with a headliner such as Frank Sinatra. There were the Paramount, the Roxy, the Strand, and in the Bronx on the Grand Concourse, the Loew's Paradise. My grandmother and I would venture out from the Bronx and get the subway train at either the 233rd Street station or the 225th Street station. She would treat me to a meal at the Horn & Hardart Automat, which was a chain of cafeterias in New York City and Philadelphia. During the 1940s and 1950s, there were more than fifty of these restaurants in New York serving over 350,000 people a day! I would usually get a hot roast beef sandwich and some pie from the glass window door.

When we moved to Yonkers, north of the city in Westchester County, I was around nine years old. I was a "latchkey kid," home for lunch by myself and home in the afternoon way before my mom and father came home from work. I had imaginary friends, imaginary games, and imaginary enemies. I never felt abandoned.

On Saturdays, my mother could get rid of me for most of the day by sending me to the local movie house, Trans Luxe, or something that sounded like that. It was three walking blocks away. For thirty-five cents, I was forgotten and orphaned. The theater was sandwiched between the neighborhood drug store and some type of general variety store. Saturday afternoons were reserved for us little brats—for a quarter, a ticket would get you an adventure serial such as *Batman* or *Flash Gordon* (usually thirteen to fourteen weeks) a cartoon, coming attractions, a movie, and usually a bad second B movie feature—often a western. My parents rarely, if ever, asked what I was seeing, and I saw films often way above my head or probably inappropriate for my age. I remember seeing *The Third Man* with my grandmother, but later alone I saw *The Rose Tattoo, A Place in the Sun, The African Queen,* and *High Noon*—all over my head. I became quite a critic, being amazingly upset when Katharine Hepburn lost to Anna Magnani for the best actress role. I was eleven or twelve, watching this film about a widowed Sicilian woman in the United States who is left damaged by the death of her husband. What the hell did I know about what was going on there?!

Often, if the movies were not good, and we went together as a group of eleven-year-old boys, this was not a good formula. I tell my children now, that I'm not proud of the things I did as a kid, and I would expect none of it from them or their kids. Some things we did as boys growing up in the Bronx were quite innocent and fun to reminisce about, like using the leftover ice cream sticks from the Good Humor man for races. We would place them in the street gutter and then pee on them to move them down the street. This may sound easy, but it was much harder than you think. In the movie house, we were boys with a different devious mission. In those days, the soda machine would drop the small plastic-coated cup, then the syrup, and finally the carbonated water. After drinking the soda, we would pee into these cups and head up to the balcony, where we would toss off these pee-filled cups upon the young audience below. We would wait for the screams, usually from the girls, and quietly go to our seats. I'm not proud—just reporting. But I did learn a lot about life from the movies—about good and evil, kissing, music influencing the emotions, the connections of lives, and even, to some degree, about courage and dignity and even dying. One could learn a lot for less than fifty cents.

As Good As It Gets

I don't recall any of my male family members ever attending regular church services, not my grandfather, father, and uncles—all Italian-American. There was no reading of the Holy Bible. My cousins and I were expected to attend Sunday Mass, receive the sacraments, and not eat meat on Fridays or all the other holy days of fast—Ash Wednesday, Good Friday, and Christmas Eve. The men in my family never seemed like spiritual folk and were anticleric, suspicious of the rules required to be a practicing Catholic. They did attend weddings and funerals as required. Of course, there were no Irish or other ethnicities of the immediate family I can name. More vowels!

My father was the third oldest of six boys and one girl, the youngest, Theresa, who was about seven years older than I. He was born in Manhattan in 1917. There had been another daughter, Anna, who died at five in the great flu pandemic of 1918. My mother was one of four. Therefore, there was an ongoing sequence of weddings and funerals of aunts, uncles, and cousins. I recall what were called "football" weddings probably in the late '40s and '50s. These happened at empty halls with round tables, each supplied with a pyramid of wax-covered sandwiches—ham, bologna, salami, etc. If your table lacked enough of what people wanted, they would "request" one from another table—which then would be tossed across to the requesting table. Such class! These events were loud and filled with the great smells of garlic, or at funerals, the horrific wails of sobbing with occasional attempts by mourners to join the dead person in the casket. Wakes would last days and end with an enormous banquet and feeding frenzy with the family—it was here that the celebration of the life remembered happened. It was the release valve and, I observed as a kid, a kind of necessary passage.

There was a dark side of the Brescia family. With so many characters, I guess it should not have been a surprise. My father's older brother, Leo, was a small, petite, and funny man. I was told he was very smart, with a gift for numbers and an awesome memory. This was useful, as he was a bookie. He could remember who had given him money for three numbers that they would bet—some in a row or just three numbers. There was never a paper trail. Unfortunately, he was a self-destructive individual, smoking heavily and drinking excessively. At age thirty-eight, he was a frequent patient at the Flower-Fifth Avenue Hospital in New York City with severe cardiovascular disease. He was no longer able to work in the soda-bottling plant and now was on New York City welfare. He and his wife, my aunt Anna, lived in a slum-like railroad apartment on East 116th Street, in the heart of Harlem. Most of the old Italians by the mid-1950s had moved up to the Bronx or to outer Queens or Long Island. The neighborhood felt old and unsafe when we would visit. The apartment had one bathroom off the kitchen with a chain to pull and flush. Anna began to run amok with known low-life criminals, and ultimately, she and her daughter, my first cousin Ann, were murdered—stabbed to death. My uncle was already dead at thirty-eight of heart disease. It was unsettling to see on the six-hour local news the bodies being removed. My father was angry, embarrassed, and upset. My cousin Anthony was sixteen at the time of his mother's and sister's murders, and he had been stabbed multiple times while trying to help save them. Anthony is still alive in the Bronx, married with two daughters and retired from the phone company. It's something we never talk about.

  I remember the strong feeling of being part of this large family, a sense of protective connection, something larger than me, and this warmth of family gave me an enormous sense of security and comfort. I thought, I am not alone, and someone cares that I am here. I don't recall much talk about religion or that the deceased family member was going to a "better place" to be with God in heaven. There was no comfort there. Grief, yes, but I never felt, at least as a kid, any great spiritual adventure to funerals. Funerals were a practical necessity. It was their time, and let's get on with it. Respect for the dead, for a family member, did matter, and the loss, we were told as kids, was forever. When my paternal grandfather, Frank, died suddenly of a massive heart attack at sixty-four, I was eleven years old. I and all my cousins were forbidden to watch television for one full year—and we followed the mandate. And after that, my grandmother never stopped wearing black.

My grandfather's sudden passing in October 1953 was the first death where I remember the feeling of sorrow and loss, experiencing the heaviness of grief. Grief, I think, is always ready to knock on the door. I realize now that it is not a medical diagnosis that can be relieved with any pill but a part of the human drama that carves away the interconnection of our lives. I would wonder—Where is he? What place has he gone to? Can he see me and hear me? Will I see my grandfather ever again? My God, this is just the beginning—someday my parents will die; someday I can and will die! At eleven, in that year of enforced mourning, I observed the patterns of behavior, remembered, and didn't ask too many questions—and I certainly didn't expect answers from this bunch of family. Death did not alter the churchgoing habits of any of my family—no one became more spiritual or ever brought up those ultimate questions concerning meaning. The religion passed on to me was formulated with rules given by my Roman Catholic catechism and was said to be the one and only truth.

The faith given to me was confusing if you really thought about it. You had to go to Mass on Sundays, and you couldn't eat meat on Fridays, or a mortal sin was committed, which, unconfessed, meant eternal damnation in hell. Riffing on this fate, comedian George Carlin noted, "But God loves you." This was quite clear to me: that all my close, loving relatives, including my parents, grandparents, uncles, and aunts—all of them were condemned and doomed to eternal punishment by this loving Jesus. Something didn't quite add up. None of the church's rules were followed by any family members.

The major holidays—Thanksgiving, Christmas, and Easter—were always taken seriously as family gathering events. On Palm Sunday we would get the "best" palms and bring them to our grandparents. Holy Thursday night we often followed a tradition of visiting three churches, and I do recall going on Good Friday to the somber stations of the cross. My mother seemed to evolve over time into a more visibly religious person—going to Mass and following the set rules. She had given up long ago on my father. The major holidays were wonderful food festivals—obviously Italian food! Meals began in the early afternoon with soup, antipasti, pasta, roast lamb or turkey, fruits, nuts, pastries, and espresso. The salad always came near the end of the meal. These adventures ended way past dark—they were magical, with the grandparents the center of gravity of the family connectedness. When it was a meatless day of obligations, no worry; a substituted feast was presented—all kinds of fish dishes, pasta with marinara or fish sauce, pizza, desserts. We never were hungry or lacked an abundance of something wonderful to eat. We were not rich, yet we never felt poor.

The Catholic faith of my Italian elders did have a magical voodoo quality. For example, the curative nature of the faith extended even to the potentially polio-infected waters of beaches in the Bronx. There was a respectable fear of getting polio if you went into polluted water, so it was avoided—except on August 8, the Feast of the Assumption of Mary, the mother of Jesus, into heaven. Somehow, on this day, the water was pure. We believed, as did our elders—somehow, they knew everything, and it all made sense (like hiding under our desks at school during a nuclear attack). There were other silly rules I questioned but obeyed, like not taking a bath for at least one half hour after eating! We prayed to the saints for deliverance from a problem and hoped the given saint would intercede for us to Jesus or the Father. I wasn't quite sure, as a kid, how all this worked. Was He too busy? Too far away?

There was a saint assigned for seemingly everything, every cause—lost causes, even. Funeral cards, given out at the wake, were saved like baseball cards with the name of the deceased and date of death. These were displayed on my grandmother's fireplace mantel, often with a candle where a proper offering could be made. The most general consistent prayer I remember was for my mother and grandmother to have a "good death," meaning to be able to die very old and quietly in their sleep without pain. As in the game Monopoly: pass go, collect $200. I observed.

My grandmother Rose died in my first year of medical school. She had rheumatic fever and heart failure over many years. I never really knew her cardiac pathology but suspect she had right-sided heart failure, with her eventual death caused by hepatic failure, ascites, jaundice, and encephalopathy. Her funeral was another where there was a need to restrain the spouse—here my grandfather—from jumping into the casket.

Grief was again knocking at the door. My grandfather was so dependent on his wife. He worked as a bootblack, shining shoes—making a good living. I never remembered my grandparents lacking for anything. He would come home in a white shirt and tie and get his bottled homemade red wine, and my grandmother would sit close as he dined, meeting his every need. Every meal had a beginning, middle, and end with a large salad, wine vinegar, black coffee, and usually some fruit. Once she was gone, eating meals lost meaning for my grandfather, and though my mother tried to take on the role of cook and waitress, it never would meet my grandfather's grief. I noticed that my paternal grandmother did better after my grandfather's death than my maternal grandfather after my grandmother's death. Men handle the loss of their spouses poorly. I would learn this fact later. My grandfather continued to work into his late seventies until a massive stroke caused his death. His great debility and poor performance state made his death seem like a blessing. Death could be a friend.

I feel, now, somewhat guilty that I didn't grieve enough at the time of my grandparents' loss. I had lived as a child in their home—I had shared meals, their lust for good food, wine, and celebrations of life. I didn't appreciate the permanence of their absence—their interconnection, their history for me of where my genes came from, the old country. The loss would be durable. Also, their loss meant having fewer people around who really knew me—what I was like as a kid, my history. Indeed, there are few who know me as I was and can correct the mistakes of my memory of the past. We die a little as those around us pass away. It's like the cosmic disappearance of the stars and galaxies as they move away from us—future generations will no longer gaze and see them.

Most of the family is gone, and by gone, I mean dead—my parents, my grandparents, all my eighteen uncles and aunts, as well as three of my twenty-one cousins. The world I lived in in the Bronx as a child, close to all these people within blocks of each other, is also long gone. It has ceased to be. The music I remember hearing also has evolved to something different, but thank goodness, the music of Sinatra that filled our home remains. Only now can I appreciate what has been lost. Indeed, I would trade all of today for what has been given up for change. I would return to my trolley ride and give up the bus. I would gladly trade my seventy-five-inch multichannel super-color television to hear again alive the theater of the mind—my radio of the 1940s—and surrender my place in any elite restaurant to smell and taste the food on my grandmother's old stove. I can only hope my children remember me with fondness when I join the parade of the family. The lesson is that it mattered, and maybe it matters more because it ceases to be, as it has to. Maybe it's the eventual potential end of things that imparts the nobility to things and events.

By the time my father died in late August 1977, I was only thirty-five. I had seen my fill of countless wakes and funerals, attended patients with incurable illnesses, watched man's inhumanity to man, and then, all at once, my dad was dead—suddenly in his sleep, one week past his sixtieth birthday. And one week after my third child, Michaelann, was born. It was the changing of the guard. One in—one out. I knew at that funeral how much I would miss him going forward. We had spoken often, two to three times each week, mostly about the nothingness of daily life—about family, my doctoring, his physical complaints, and always about what was happening with the family. Family was everything to his life, and it was a major reason why I stayed close to home for my medical training. That's all I knew as well. Events in one's life do change the landscape of how we see the world and ourselves. My grandmother, my growing up in the Bronx of the 1940s, my Italian American culture, Vietnam, and now my father's death—it was like now I was the adult in a serious adult world. I now would become a better observer, if nothing else. Life should be looked at with some effort to funnel meaning and reverence into my life. I also was next—I had to figure stuff out.

On my sixty-fifth birthday, I was given a surprise party by my wife, Jane, who invited close family and lifelong friends. We celebrated dinner at the Redeye Grill on West Fifty-Sixth and Seventh Avenue, directly across from Carnegie Hall in New York. As a gift, I received an honorary high school diploma from Mount Saint Michael Academy, an all-boys Catholic prep school in the Bronx that had rejected my application three separate times—in sixth grade, seventh grade, and ninth grade. This honor was a concatenation of my wife and my childhood friend John Farrauto, who was on the board of trustees of the school. Both Jane and John had known my long-winded rants against the school, in which I noted that it had rejected a future physician and generally good person. I really disliked the Mount.

Mount Saint Michael Academy was located in the Wakefield neighborhood of the Bronx, close to where I grew up, on the border of Westchester County. At the time I applied, it was located on a twenty-two-acre campus and run by the Marist Brothers of the Catholic Church. My friends were going there, some in grammar school and later some in high school. I was defeated three times, rejected for the sixth-grade class, seventh-grade class, and high school. The first rejection was very personal: I failed a one-on-one interview and question session with an elderly Marist brother. I certainly must have come across with little flair or hope for any academic future. It's hard to remember oneself at a particular time and place. I can envision the large room with old wooden floors and bookcases and a large overpowering desk. I remember a smell of old wood. I remember the lighting needing some help. I don't recall the questions. I don't remember anything more than the man's somber, unfriendly demeanor. I can't remember if I was dismissed on the spot and spared a letter of rejection or if I had to wait for the humiliation.

This event was repeated a second time—a year later, with the same outcome. I remember the second rejection well, and I don't know why. I see myself alone in my paternal grandparents' apartment, near a window and sobbing uncontrollably. I felt stupid, alone, and angry. The last rejection wasn't so personal—this time I failed a generalized admission computer test. At least I wasn't a witness to my rejector. By this time, I was accustomed to rejection from many schools. I didn't cry, but I was still angry. However, I was a little older and somehow began to sense I had some ownership in my stupidity. There was something brewing within me for the first time that acknowledged my part in all this—my laziness. I also began over time to understand that this need came from within me—but I hated the Mount!

The multiple rejections from Mount Saint Michael Academy became an awakening and an internal rally cry for me. I really now believe that the experience of not attending the Mount was saying that what could have been was better than if I had been accepted. But going "up the ladder" and doing well was, for me, attached to a sense of inferiority—there was always a question about self-doubt or seeing something in myself that others could not see. I have heard this same idea from close friends with successful medical careers who attended foreign medical schools because of rejection from American medical schools. How often we assume so wrongly about others and ourselves! I had won the pursuit I had sought and struggled to succeed in. Sometimes you can see things in life only in reverse.

I was headed for public high school—and that probably would have worked out well. By high school, I was motivated. I wanted to be a physician. One of my neighborhood friends suggested we take the entrance exam for Sacred Heart High School in Yonkers. It was coeducational, meaning girls, and it was growing from a small parish school to a larger regional high school. I'm convinced I passed because they needed students to fill the desks. Tuition was twelve dollars each month—affordable for my parents. I was accepted. The school needed me, but in truth, I really needed it more. My first year in high school was the most difficult academic year I have ever had. I had to learn how to learn—to become a real student. It's a matter of understanding what's important and what's not. That year was harder than premed at Fordham and, I would think, even medical school.

Somewhere in my last year of elementary school, I took an anatomy course—cut open a frog. I remember my grandmother, when cooking, would make a point of showing me the organs of the animal we were having for dinner—"This is the liver, intestines, and lungs." She had a zeal for showing me the importance of the animal parts and explained carefully and simply to me what she knew these organs actually did. No other members of my family ever shared anything more of themselves than this woman born of poor farmers in Italy. I wonder now if she was showing off her craft as a superb chef, or was it something more—was she seeing something in me for the future? Probably not, but I do sometimes wonder if she was preparing my future. I remember her slaughtering a pig in our backyard in the Bronx. I don't recall that I was upset or repelled by the act. Food was food, and it was the dead animal sacrificed for a purpose. I must confess I never hunted, and I never missed the shooting opportunity. My grandmother would often take me to get a chicken freshly killed on the site of a Bronx slaughterhouse. Emotions are infectious to little kids, and I detected no attachment of my grandmother to the anatomies of my food. I saw no personal connection to the liver or spleen that was being prepared for a meal. There is a difference between dissecting the organs of a cadaver, I learned later as a medical student, and cutting up a chicken to eat. And we Italians ate all the organs. Nothing was ever wasted—stomachs, testicles, brains.

I don't know the reasoning that suddenly motivated me to try harder when I reached high school. But, I wanted to be someone who mattered, who made a difference—a doctor. With that decision, I needed good—no, excellent—grades to attend a reputable college that would get me accepted to an American medical school. The competition was fierce. My father, interestingly, became a huge cheerleader for me. This, I learned, was an important opportunity—not so much for me as an individual but for the family! Nothing would bring more immediate respect to me, my father, and the family as a whole than to have a physician in the family. How great America must have seemed to my grandparents—here, in one generation, after coming from the poorest area of Italy, to have a physician among us. It is a testimony to the United States, how we allow opportunity to those who strive and work hard. Indeed, even if I had become a physician and tried to go back to the old country to practice medicine, the Italians would have still seen me as a product of a family that were farmers, poor, and unable to make it there. Little Frankie—a doctor.

My mindset was like that of many of my peers who also chose to be doctors. I had become super focused as I entered premed at Fordham University at age seventeen. My eye was on the prize of medical school. Fifty young men were accepted into the pre-medical program and the university somewhat hinted that if we got through the rigorous studies and received a general recommendation from Fordham, we most likely would get accepted to an American medical school. This was a big deal. I worked my ass off, and one begins to sacrifice fun times for a romance of study and achievement and most of all good grades: As and B-pluses. I was accepted to medical school early in the fall of my senior year of college, and my MCAT scores made the grade. I was on my way. I had no serious girlfriend.

In late August, a month prior to starting medical school, I was trying to get a date with a neighborhood girl I suddenly fancied—Rosary was her first name. It was a dark, clear summer night, and I went to her home. Nobody was around—all dark. I walked the several blocks home and noticed a strange car in the driveway. It was reasonably late, nine thirtyish for usual visitors to our house. Small beginnings, the timing of vague happenings, and everything in one's life changes. My father's old friend from grammar school and his wife were near the neighborhood, and they had decided to stop by with their daughter Marjorie. I had known of the Di Marco family through conversations my parents had with my grandparents. They seemed to know all about one another. This was a "good" Italian family.

I came home and was introduced. It didn't seem like anyone was moving, so I suggested Marjorie and I go out to watch the horse race at the Yonkers Raceway not too far away. It was reasonably pleasant. The next days, apparently, were notable for conversations between Mike, who was Marjorie's father, and my dad. And finally, the query, "Why don't you ask her out? They are a good family." I was much too weak and tired to fight this kind of pressure, and I succumbed. It's hard to believe the pressure families will place on their offspring to keep the genetic code limited! I had dated in college a very pleasant girl from the Bronx—Rosemary Brandi. As it turned out, she was in the same Hunter College class as Marjorie. Apparently, Rosemary was not a "good choice" for me. She was Italian American—yes. However, her family came from northern Italy—Alta Italia—and her family did not speak like us, and more importantly, they did not cook like us. They used cream sauces in their food. That was a real hindrance to romance!

I really was not too bright. Being a doctor was the only goal and end point. Settling down and getting married, which was expected, was of secondary importance. I'm making awful excuses for what happened—I got married in my second year of medical school! Medical school leaves little time for deep social and marital connections. Internship and residency were even more demanding and inhibitory to my forming a better relationship. I then went to Vietnam and completed a medical oncology fellowship at Memorial Sloan Kettering Cancer Center (MSKCC). Our first child was born eight years after we were married. No foundation of a life truly was established. I was too young and too stupid to have married at twenty-three. It was really never fair to either of us to expect anything more than what happened. Her father, Mike, had been diagnosed with advanced colon cancer near the time they visited my parents. Marjorie's mother never told Mike or her that she knew that he would die of this illness. Our wedding plans were moved up to have him there, but it was sad and tragic. He was frail and ill appearing confined to a wheelchair, and dead less than three months later. Death had another role to play in life.

Some things are destined to be or need to happen. My four children from this marriage bring joy and value to both Marjorie's and my lives. I would want it no other way. I see both of us in them. What if I had found that girl I was seeking that August night? What if I had gotten home too late? What if I had said no to my father—"You take her out"? What if I had just dated her and moved on without committing? How much say did I even have here? Of note, as an aside, my father regretted I married his friend's daughter, but that was before he got to know his grandchildren. I was twenty three years old. I had no business being married.

You question yourself after a marriage dies. Who are you? My priorities were simply off! And you do come to the realization of how much we really change in life—our motivations, our desires, our likes and dislikes, our expectations about people and the future. Always looking at tomorrow. And above all, you learn about the meaning of people in your life. My son, Frankie, for a long time dated and lived with a very smart young woman with a depressive personality. After spending a few minutes with her, you needed to stay away from all sharp instruments. Her downer mood had become infectious to those around her. This had an especially noticeable effect on my son's personality. After several years of watching this, I finally told Jane I needed to say something, and I did. "Frankie, it is none of my business if you want to continue to stay and even marry this woman. But if you are thinking that way, the question you need to ask yourself is whether she is what you want to see first thing each and every future morning. If so, go for it, but if not, then run!" Within the next two months, somehow it was finally over. And more than this—when he did finally meet someone new and marry, he toasted her on their wedding day with "I can't wait to wake up each day and see you there!" Sometimes, you know as a parent that you got it near right. It is always, always, about our tomorrows!

PART II:
Becoming a Doctor

Medical school happens quickly. Maybe the reason the four years of medical school go so fast is that the years preparing to get in are so hard and filled with anxiety and doubt. In a brief four years, and still at the young age of twenty-five, one becomes a physician. Getting into medical school always seemed like an end point, but it was the starting point. No longer a layperson, you are now called "Doctor." It is assumed you know a lot more than you do; it is assumed that you're dedicated, hardworking, ethical, compassionate, and intelligent. Truly becoming a physician demands time. Time to study, time to practice a craft, time to know your patients in the best and worst of their lives, time to take examinations and more examinations, time to be reviewed and watched, time to learn it again, all over again. The word is *sacrifice*. Sacrifice your sleep, sacrifice your relationships, sacrifice holidays. Sacrifice your health. Become observant. Think critically. Watch your teachers. Practice. Gain experience. Learn how to communicate with simple language. Don't be afraid of smells and blood and nasty stuff. Ask questions. Admit mistakes. Show humility.

Smile sometimes. Listen to nurses. Think about pain and suffering. Watch and heal the dying. Speak to families. Touch the ill. See each patient as Adam, the first man. Know your place. Become the teacher and mentor you wanted. Know what it means to be the good and noble physician.

    You are greeted the first day of class in medical school with death. Lessons of medicine begin with the close of life, with the presentation of a cadaver. We all knew this was coming—the anxiety about passing multiple hard courses and meeting a dead body. There was the distinct smell of formalin embalming that filled the room on the twelfth floor of the basic science building of my school—Seton Hall College of Medicine, later to become a state school under the Rutgers umbrella. I met the new classmates who would join me as cadaver dissection partners—Andy Guay, Paula Kraft. We met our dead woman—an elderly white-haired lady. There was a soberness to this meeting—a solemn initiation into the world of doctoring. We young students would be transformed by this woman as we dissected respectfully into this body. Our job would be to know her anatomy well—where blood flows and veins and nerves cross. It would be about relationships so that one day in the future I would insert a large needle into something of bodily importance and not cause harm. Hours would be invested into cutting carefully, watching every movement of the scalpel to avoid damaging or distorting organs. We moved slowly, with cautious deliberation. We dissected at awful hours—the cadaver laboratory was kept open to enable us to finish our work. And we were tired—so tired that we no longer talked about it. No one outside this room even cared, and besides, this was what we had signed up for. No person outside this world could imagine what the hell we were doing anyway—11:00 p.m., cold outside, pizza box open, dissecting a woman's corpse with the smell of formaldehyde and death all around. Are you kidding me?

    Midyear into anatomy, about the time we had reached the lower extremity, I realized that my lady cadaver's leg was not properly "fixated," or embalmed correctly. The leg was a mush of tissue unable to be separated by a knife. I could not learn anatomy on this body's lower leg. What was I to do? There were graduate anatomy students who, with the faculty, helped guide us. "My cadaver's leg is unable to be dissected as is." The fix was for me to get a new leg. In the bowels of the Jersey City Medical Canter—a monstrous hospital building that housed one thousand beds—was the place where the cadavers were kept. "Go get a new leg" was the instruction. I must confess, I really wasn't quite sure what that all meant at the time. I asked a classmate, Mike Debella, to come with me. He was a funny guy who would wear colorful polka-dot underwear trunks that would show brightly through the white pants we wore as students.

The medical center was huge, built by the Jersey City Democratic machine during the Depression. There was a famous maternity hospital, the Margaret Hague, and a respiratory center hospital where Sister Kenney worked against polio for children in iron lungs. The directions must have been good because I don't recall having trouble finding the place. The basement of the medical center was large—and by *large*, I mean one could drive a trailer truck on this highway belowground. There was an anteroom we entered where three corpses hung in the corner. This, I recall, was the place where the 1930 Frankenstein horror movies must have been made. I remember an attendant telling me, after handing me a hacksaw, to go through another door, which would lead me to the bodies. "Take what you need—a leg, isn't it?"

This room we entered was an enormous warehouse-like cathedral—well lit, very cold, but with a couple of hundred bodies hanging as in a meat market. The floor was moist—even wet—with a light slimy red-pink tincture. I thought, Holy shit!! They must be fucking kidding me! But I do need a leg! How desperate am I? There were nervous, anxious—holy shit—giggles. Mike wanted no part of the amputation—this was all my show. I chose. I never looked up at the corpse I had decided to mutilate. I took my hacksaw and began the awful deed. I forced the saw through the bone, and as I remember, the task was more difficult because the body was hanging by the neck very high off the ground. When done, I placed what I had severed into a white towel I had taken and walked back through the hospital lobby carrying a leg to my cadaver lab. It was done.

There were no celebrations when my dead lady was finally totally unrecognizable as a past person. I do remember being with her the last time and thanking her for her gift to us. I know nothing more about this woman. There was no life—no soul to dissect. At the time I wondered if she could witness my progress and my tiredness, as well as my frustration of needing to know so much that I would forget. I do not know how she died. I do not know if she had a happy childhood or a good life. I do not know if she was missed or even if she is missed now. I do not know any more about life, where it goes, or what meaning she offered. All I can measure are her parts. But I wish, somehow, she could know how she helped me go from being an unknowing person to being a physician. You suddenly realize how much society gives to you—to know intimate details about people. Society allows you to touch them, to probe and give advice.

I can't recall my first patient death in medical school. Perhaps I was too tired or too young to comprehend the gravity of the situation. Maybe I should have been more reflective about what I was seeing—the distractions around patient illness, the families, their loss of ability to work, their ongoing pain, their sadness and depression, their suffering. We needed to know facts and relationships of facts. We needed to connect anatomy with pathology and biochemistry with physiology and microbiology, statistical possibilities with this or that complaint. Death was the enemy, and we were there to confront and stop it. There were no courses given on the humanity of illness or of breaking bad news, none on relieving pain and less on recognizing suffering, and nothing about the meaning of death. These were so-called soft topics. I think everyone in my medical school class felt a void in our education. I certainly did—and maybe my Jesuit Fordham philosophy stuff was beginning to show its ugly head. One starts to think!

Even though I had honor grades in surgery, I hated the confines of surgery and the limitations of OB-GYN practice at that time. Neurology seemed an intellectual sport with little gain in patient improvement. I saw orthopedics as anatomical carpentry and urology as nonintellectual anatomical plumbing. I had thought psychiatry was a possible outcome for me, but all my medical school teachers seemed *"pazzo "(crazy)*, as my grandmother would say. Mothers made me give up on pediatrics. I needed to engage with people and therefore left pathology and radiology to my nonspeaking friends. Dermatology was a good possibility, but I sensed I needed more. And there was internal medicine—I could be a "real doctor," a diagnostician, something like the catcher on a baseball team, seeing the whole game all at once. Was I smart or observant enough to put the connections together?

We lacked any real oncology exposure in medical school. But to be exact, there was little that was known or could be done for many of the cancers in the late fifties and early sixties. There was one oncologist on my medical school faculty, a doctor who, fifteen years later, unfortunately, became my patient. This internal urge about general medicine and the obvious newness of the branch of medicine termed medical oncology seemed promising to me. Most malignancies (leukemia, lymphomas, Hodgkin's disease) were managed by hematologists or general surgeons who appeared comfortable using the limited drugs available. I placed as my number one choice for internship the Cornell program, which listed a three-month requirement at Memorial Sloan Kettering Cancer Center ("MSKCC"), on Sixty-Seventh and Sixty-Eighth Streets, from First Avenue to York Avenue in Manhattan. Across the street were New York Hospital, Hospital for Special Surgery, Rockefeller Hospital, and Cornell Medical School. The Sloan Kettering Research Center was next door as well.

I had broken the Mount Saint Michael Academy curse. I was one of twelve straight medicine interns—half having graduated from Cornell Medical School and the others from Jefferson, Georgetown, and Indiana. This was a really bright group of people. And indeed, over the next years, I met more bright young physicians—they would become chairs of departments and directors of cancer centers. Then there was me. I realized it was better to be the least smart—I learned so much.

In 1968, the Cornell Medical division moved out of Bellevue Hospital in New York, as did the Columbia Medical School division, which moved to Harlem Hospital. Only New York University Medical School stayed. My mentors had all been Bellevue Hospital physicians and were now at North Shore University Hospital in Manhasset, on Long Island. I would do nine months there, three months at Memorial during my internship year, and four months at Memorial during my first year of residency. The prestigious, competitive residency programs paid less and had you work harder. "Every other night" meant being on call Monday, Wednesday, Saturday, Sunday, Tuesday, Thursday, and Friday. I once was on call from 8:00 a.m. Saturday until 5:00 p.m. Tuesday. This was before residency work rules were established by the Bell Commission in New York. It was not unheard of to get eight admissions in one day. I was chronically tired, married, and learning to be a good physician—my initial goal. I had sacrificed a great deal, but there, through all this, it gave me an internal sense of pride—that I could do this with the best of the best.

Suddenly, your life and dreams begin. My internship began July 1, 1968. I had matched to the Cornell University program—that program recently, along with Columbia, had left Bellevue Hospital. We would be required to spend three months at Memorial Sloan Kettering Cancer Center and the James Ewing Hospital for Cancer in New York City. I was excited! I stayed for another year and applied for the fellowship program in medical oncology at Memorial Hospital. It was a transition time for cancer treatment and training. Treatment was no longer just radical surgery; the field underwent a paradigm shift to recognizing that this was a systemic illness and you couldn't just cut it out and expect things to get better. Memorial was at the center of novel thinking—understanding mechanisms of cancer biology, immune modulators, target sites, better supportive measures, pain management, and psychosocial options. I was to be a medical oncologist with a new medical board recognizing this specialty. I was in the second group to take the medical oncology board examination.

I felt I belonged. Gifted people became my teachers. Smart people were all around me—faculty, residents, fellows in training, medical students, and specialized nurses. The place had a long history filled with tradition and the legacies of former pioneers in cancer medicine. And they were interested in making me a better physician. Oncology filled what I was seeking—newness of a specialty—and I was at ground level. There would be constant change, with novel ideas, medicines, and paradigm shifts. I could and must deal with multiple specialties, patients young and old, and added questions from patients given to us to solve—psychosocial, spiritual, suffering-related, and economic. I would have to face my old friends' grief and loss and think about God's role in all this. And I was around really talented, smart people who wanted to nourish me—what could be better? Plus, I was in my most favorite world—New York!

The Vietnam War had been raging when I had graduated from medical school in June 1968. It had been a turbulent year. That March, in medical school, acting as an extern in my fourth year, I was at Martland Newark City Hospital the night that Martin Luther King Jr. was assassinated—I had a hard time getting home through the riots that followed. Robert Kennedy was also killed that June. There was unrest. I just wanted to get through my training. I knew I would be drafted to go to 'Nam. They needed physicians. I decided to enlist via the Berry Plan—an option which a physician committed to service but by lottery could hope to get enough time to complete training and also select a branch of service. I requested five years for medical oncology completion and the navy. I was anticipating the war would be over. I was given one year and the US Army. My orders came in the spring of 1970—Vietnam. I was to report in November in San Francisco. I was off to war! Academic residencies and fellowships go from July through June each year. This order to start in November meant I had no academic job, no place to live, and no health-care benefits for four months. Thank you, army! Memorial accepted my application for the medical oncology fellowship when I completed my two-year commitment to the army. I was married without any children.

PART III:
Learning about Caring for the Dying

Calvary Hospital is the only acute care hospital in the country that cares for people exclusively with limited life expectancy and a need for hospitalization. It is located in the northeast section of the Bronx and has two hundred beds. It has a full-time medical staff and a remarkable history of delivering excellent end-of-life care. Its history dates back to the start of the last century, when nine women in lower Manhattan began to care for poor dying women. It was managed by a religious order of Catholic nuns and was later taken over by the Catholic Archdiocese of New York.

In 1970, as I finished my second year of residency in New York at the Cornell University Hospitals, I had my orders for Vietnam. At that time, Calvary was located in a poor section of the South Bronx, near the Jerome Avenue elevated subway line. The good sisters were the nurses and administrators, and there were only one hundred beds. It was a place to die. Many of the dying were poor. It had recently become accredited as a hospital. The sisters had persuaded a few physicians to volunteer their time and then later persuaded them to come on full time.

The medical director was Dr. James Cimino. He was known as Jack. Jack was an incredibly gifted physician with high standards of what it meant to be a physician—all about nonabandonment. He, with my cousin Michael Brescia, the son of my grandfather Frank's brother Louis, became full time. These two physicians were well known in nephrology, having conceived of an arteriovenous shunt (the Cimino-Brescia) to help solve the problem of access to blood vessels for hemodialysis. This was a major medical discovery. A seminal paper on this topic grew out of their work at the Bronx Veterans Hospital and was published in the *New England Journal of Medicine* in 1966. They brought in several other physicians to become part of the hospital's first full-time staff—interestingly, all Italian-American: Dr. Eufemio, Dr. Riario, and Dr. Briamante. Dr. Cimino died of cancer in 2010, and my cousin Michael Brescia died in April 2023 at age ninety.

Because Calvary was now a specialized hospital, it required medical coverage at night. It paid well, hourly, and the work was not too difficult—mostly pronouncing and filling out death certificates. Occasionally, there was a fever workup, a pain crisis, or a need to evaluate a change in a patient's condition. I was in my second year of internal medicine training at Cornell in 1970 with orders to leave for Vietnam in early November. Several of the senior residents and even faculty at Memorial Sloan Kettering worked moonlighting up in the South Bronx. Karl Adler, who was my chief resident that year, worked one night each week. I knew I needed a job for at least four months after June 1970, so I called Michael and tested the waters. The hospital needed extra night coverage that spring and would hire me for full-time work after July into November.

Memorial Hospital is on the plush East Side of Manhattan, between Sixty-Seventh and Sixty-Eighth Streets and cornered by First Avenue and York, close to the East River. The new hospital had just opened near the new clinic building on Sixty-Eighth Street. We lived, as did many interns, residents, and fellows, in the apartments across the street. It was an easy walking commute. The city bus stopped at the corner and would take you through the park to Lincoln Center. The neighborhood had many restaurants, particularly on First Avenue. It was an ideal location to live and learn.

I committed to work Tuesday nights at Calvary up in the Bronx. The Jerome Avenue IRT line would get me there from Manhattan within an hour. This was the train that passed Yankee Stadium and often could be seen on the Yankees' televised games. I believe it was the Mount Eden station where I exited. I was really anxious on my first trip to work at Calvary. I wasn't sure what to expect. The neighborhood was not the ritzy East Side of Manhattan—this was the South Bronx. Buildings were old, and they looked old. No carnival atmosphere here for my first visit. I remember it was on Featherbed Lane—someone suggested it was given that name because of houses of prostitution there. Don't quote me on that one. The hospital looked nothing like a hospital. It was a large redbrick fortress that had a wall around the building. I was surprised it was on a hill. That section of the Bronx on the southern west side was high and impressive. There was no activity surrounding the building. The neighborhood was quiet, with very little parading of pedestrians or children playing outside. There was an open area where I assumed deliveries were made and ambulances brought patients in and where hearses would remove the dead.

This was indeed a place where the poor and dying went. I was struck, as I went inside the House of Calvary, as it was called, with the sense of peace and quiet that prevailed. No loudspeaker calling off doctors' names. No clatter of trays was heard. And above all, I noted no smells. A sister in a full black habit greeted me, smiling, and was obviously happy I had come.

My room was small, with a bed, TV, and bathroom. I do remember a window and a phone. I would work until 7:00 a.m. at Calvary Hospital and then, return to work back at

Memorial. My job here was to make the dying more comfortable—to relieve their pain and speak to their families if there was a chance—but there was no code blue here. Everyone here was prepared for death and a spiritual return to our maker. I would face no conflict with options or choices. The patients' hope here was to get to heaven.

Downtown, at Memorial, I was learning to become a medical oncologist—a cancer specialist—at the best cancer hospital in the country. The mission was to solve the mystery of a disease in the most scientific, rigorous way. In the Bronx, I was to accept defeat, understand pain, and be present for the inevitable. I was seeing life and illness and medicine's full arena. I was to learn from simple sisters of the sick and poor about nonabandonment for people I no longer could cure.

I was to learn about doctoring—become the good doctor. It was an enviable position to be in as a student of medicine—seeing it from both sides and learning from the masters of science at Memorial and the doctors of compassion at Calvary. And to my surprise, the lessons of their wisdom have stayed with me. To care for the dying doesn't require less of you as a physician; it demands much more. The lesson was to be a better clinician, a better listener, and really understand the ultimate goals of my care. What then was passed on to me? I thought about what I had been taught.

Patients do embrace their frightening reality and finality while holding on to those small scraps of hope (things might be better tomorrow than today) that make life worth living. There is no argument that the remaining quality of life for those that are dying actively is dependent on the care and decisions and options offered in the final phase of management. In this era of fewer people dying at home and fewer people witnessing death, the anticipation of some dramatic deathbed scene fills families' and patients' imaginations. Enough people die on television and in movies in melodramatic ways to make us all quite nervous. Sometimes, both the patient and the patient's family need to find a scapegoat to relieve their negative images, while the caregivers themselves may see criticisms as personal attacks on their competency and integrity.

What do dying patients worry most about? Often, they are very silent—but they usually want to die with some so-called dignity. Truly, they don't want to die at all. The primary distress for these patients often relates to unacceptable symptoms, unrelieved pain, and added unnecessary suffering in an environment of health delivery that is costly, toxic, inconvenient, and impersonal. People need explanations and advice about what may or could or probably will or will not happen as the disease progresses. Sometimes patients want no involvement; talk to my caregiver and leave me the hell out of this. But somebody should know something. Especially if the goal is to stay at home or receive some sign about when hospitalization is needed. Each potential problem near the end may need to be discussed so fears and inadequacies of the patient's treatment are placed into perspective. Every effort should be made to ascertain whether or not people are uncomfortable, even when they cannot or do not express themselves. Simple things include improving measures of physical comfort by simply changing positioning, suctioning excessive saliva, giving back rubs, and providing appropriate grooming. This advocacy must be considered to allow the dying individual to feel dignified and presentable for visitors, procedures, and examinations. To be made to feel like a member of the human community. All that can appropriately be done medically must and should be considered, while unnecessary procedures, tests, and treatments that only create added anxiety should be avoided, despite medical acceptability, reimbursement, assurance, or investigational motivation. The clinical status should always be discussed with other health-care team members, including other physicians and consultants, so that all suggestions for alleviating symptoms are given serious thought.

The philosophy of good care mandates accountability and continuity. There should be no breaks in who is treating a patient, and there should be a real sense of advocacy for patients' needs—patients should feel that the caregivers are troubled by their troubles. In the Bronx vernacular: patients want to know that someone gives a shit about them. The care plan should be documented so that all those involved in the management have clear, correct, and precise understanding of the standing orders, as well as who will be responsible for supervision and accountable for decisions. Patients often lose their capacity to decide on next steps, and loved ones may either feel guilty for the patients' deaths if they sense not enough was done, or, at the other end, feel responsible for their loved ones' continued suffering if they sought more treatment. Never quite easy.

People should be afforded every opportunity to discuss their diagnoses, prognoses, options, and costs of care in terms they can understand. The privacy of such conversations is paramount, and confidentiality must always be respected—their confidences must be kept like the confessions heard by a priest, never shared for the sake of gossip.

Patients need to have their emotional and psychological needs attended to, whether these involve worsening anxiety, depression, or problems related to the adjustment to what's happening to them. Some patients, indeed, may have long-standing mental illnesses, which may add to the challenge. Staff should strive to accept the patients' defenses and not react to these in a way that patients may feel as rejection. Many painful, distressing psychiatric symptoms may be exhibited during the last week and days of a long illness. Unfortunately, inexperienced or impotent oncology staff may lack information about common psychiatric syndromes and fail to use appropriate psychotropic medication. Appropriate patient acceptance of their fate, albeit with true sadness for loss, must be distinguished from true clinical depression. Calling a psychiatric consultation may be meaningful, but usually, patients frown about the stigma it represents along with the cost and inconvenience of seeing another doctor.

The relatives of dying patients can make the situation easier—and sometimes they can create their own hell, if not purgatory. Families need to be respected and given time for communication to allow comprehension of what's happening, grieving, and finally closure. They can offer so much insight into your patient's background and history—often completing the narrative that seemed to be missing. I've learned so much about my patients through talking with family members. What great lives they have lived! But no longer is there the hope of future promises, but perhaps the regretful sighs of a multitude of unmet dreams—the awful reflection of what could have been. Guilt, bitterness, and regret about something long past often make relationships problematic near the end. The roles of family members may be reversed, especially as the cognitive ability of the patient deteriorates. The child becomes the parent. A younger brother now must be the one to be looked up to. In all this, family and loved ones usually wish to be kept up to date, be informed of change, be at the bedside near death, and hopefully be given the opportunity to share the last words of their story—the end of an epic novel.

I realized that spiritual needs also must be considered for the dying. Often, spiritual comforts are the most crucial and important of all their wants. Religious beliefs are not necessary to instill or obligatory to foster at this time. As George Carlin noted—not the time to read the Holy Book as if cramming for a final exam! Some patients die incredibly fearful of past unforgiven sins that they have kept close to them. One of my patients, weeks away from dying, each night was dreaming she was burning in hell. This is no way to die, and we needed practical spiritual advice to help this elderly woman, who had sinned profoundly in her mind. In the end, the team of clergy and religious women helped her find peace. Among the bereaved, religiosity may be predictive not of distress but of the ability to seek help. In those studies where dying respondents stated they were religious, they appeared to self-report less depression, anxiety, or frustration.

As a physician, I, too, must be watchful of my own condition and demeanor. Practicing oncology is a medical experience of facing continuing losses that may translate feelings of helplessness in the caregiver to actions of helplessness. I may feel helpless—I cannot act helpless. So I must watch for the arousal of distressful feelings such as frustration, anger, sadness, and a sense of failure in myself. These, if left unrecognized, can be self-destructive. The caregiver must observe, feel, sense, and know his/her patient and be concerned, yet at a safe distance.

Clinicians must guard against the inevitable natural consequences of both their clinical and their personal behavior with patients and their loved ones: (1) over involvement with patients (burnout), (2) lack of involvement (cynical distraction), (3) avoidance, and (4) personal stress behavior (mood changes, alcohol, drugs, marital conflict, suicide). Noted surgeon Balfour Mount wrote about this years ago—when we are facing our losses, these feelings must not be hidden because they motivate behavior in a negative way. His suggestions are useful: seek openness of goals, be flexible with team decision-making, ensure away time and diversional activities, and seek feedback from others.

Finally, I confess that often the terminal person becomes different because we clinicians treat the person very differently—many times with apathy and indifference, not to mention with incompetency. We can refuse to address the frustration of feeling the failure of continual loss, and the caregivers can become victims of their own technology and inventiveness, ordering tests and futile treatments in a failing cause. Ultimately, it's my presence and concern that matter. No matter how much more time is actually left for a patient or how meaningful a response the patient has to a novel cancer treatment, those left behind remember the issues that really matter: How much pain and suffering was there? Was compassion shown during the dark days? Did medical professionals communicate so that loved ones understood what was going on? Did medical professionals care, and were they troubled like they promised? This clinical presence becomes the real and only important principle: nonabandonment. And I wonder—how often have I failed this test?

I learned an enormous amount about being a complete physician in those early months working with the sisters of the sick and poor. This was a special place in one of the poorest parts of the city, a place taking care of the poorest and sickest of us. People, often without family and with few options during their last days, would die here. I would often see patients treated at Memorial and then sent to Calvary to die, and I would notice how much "better" and more comfortable they appeared. There were no malodors or cries in the night of anguish or pain. There seemed in this old building in the South Bronx to be peace, comfort, calmness, and closure. One particular sister, Amata Galligan, would sit knitting dolls at dying patients' bedsides so they would not be alone when they met God. The dolls would be sold as gifts in the small gift store. When a patient died, I remember the respect in getting the body ready and leaving the room empty for a day so the soul would have time to leave. This was also a place to gather one's life and save one's soul. This sister, by the way, who would not abandon her patients, had dedicated her life to God since surviving the sinking of the *Lusitania* in 1915. What gifts life can bring forth. I observed. For many patients, sick and suffering, it seemed at times to be the most meaningful part of their lives. How is that possible? I asked myself.

In December 1980, I became the medical director of Calvary Hospital. The place had since moved to the Northeast Bronx, to a small campus across from the Albert Einstein College of Medicine. Jack had decided to give up as medical director and persuaded me to leave my practice as a medical oncologist. My life and work would be altered for a time. I stayed for fifteen years.

A word about this saintly woman, Amata, whom I would see walking the halls at night, sitting at the bedside of someone dying so that person would not be alone. She was born in Ireland in 1893, Her original name, Margaret, was from Ardlougher, Ballinagh, in County Cavan, Ireland. She and her aunt Bridget Lee were second-class passengers coming to the United States on the *Lusitania*. The two of them had planned to take the *Cameronia* across the Atlantic, but the ship's requisitioning by the British admiralty reshuffled them to the *Lusitania*. Margaret and her aunt were 2 of 766 survivors of the German U-boat attack in 1915. She was sitting and having lunch on May 7, 1915, when the ship was torpedoed by a German U-boat. There was a second explosion, and she and her aunt held each other as the ship went down. They held on to a floating deck chair for two hours before they were picked up in a lifeboat for twenty people. Margaret promised to devote her life to God if saved and in 1918 entered the Dominican Sisters of the Sick Poor. She worked at Calvary for the last fifteen years of her life and died at age seventy-nine in 1973.

PART IV:
Vietnam

I did go to Vietnam that early November 1970, after completing six weeks of jungle training in San Antonio at Fort Sam Houston, learning to become an army captain, a battalion surgeon. I was able to experience things like tear gas up close, undergo live ammunition fire, crawl through barbed wire, and shoot an M16 rifle at a target—which I must admit I never hit. I realized how protected a life I had lived before all this. I was a kid from the Bronx. I was never a Boy Scout. I never camped outside in the woods. I was never west of West Orange, New Jersey. I had never handled or shot a gun before. I had never flown on an airplane. The Bronx had always been my home. My family were city people. All at once, or at least in six weeks, I was an army captain, headed off to the Far East to be in a real war. They even gave me a .45-caliber pistol! Were these people crazy!? Despite my severe nearsightedness, I was going—what if I broke my glasses? No help there. The army offered me a chance to delay my deployment to Vietnam to join the Special Forces in Panama, where I could really learn jungle training and parachute out of planes. I declined.

As Good As It Gets

I arrived in Bien Hoa, Vietnam, and was assigned as a battalion surgeon to the First Brigade, Fifth Infantry Division stationed in the northern sector of Vietnam, Quang Tri. There were approximately one thousand soldiers here in this unit, and I was the new doctor. I now saw death and dying in a new and different way. Unlike in my residency, this time dying was not from an illness or a genetic mistake, nor was it from a terrible accident. This was not because of an individual's poor and reckless choices or bad habits like smoking and excessive alcohol consumption. This was simply collective human insanity. My own death was a strong possibility. It was as if I had been transported to another planet—another time and climate, with a new language of military talk, without control to go where I wanted, when I wanted to go. No dress options. Nothing was familiar, and I was very distant from all those I loved.

Bien Hoa was one of the oldest cities in South Vietnam. The French had conquered it in 1861 after a protracted resistance. During the Vietnam conflict when I was there, it was a major US Air Force base and from where I would receive my final orders for duty. I was there four or five days before learning I had been assigned as the battalion surgeon to the infantry division in the northern part of the country, Quang Tri. Quang Tri was twelve miles south of North Vietnam and three miles from Laos, where the Ho Chi Minh Trail was. I didn't know it at the time of my arrival in November 1970, but I would be part of the Lam Son invasion in February 1971, which would kill five thousand South Vietnamese troops. I would take care of some of those casualties.

The rainy season in the northern part of the country was about to begin as I arrived, making traveling from Bien Hoa a challenge because the airstrips would be flooded and underwater. My plane would attempt a landing and halfway to my destination return me back to Da Nang, which was the first stop off from Bien Hoa. Rain was followed by more rain. The Da Nang airport was not JFK, and I slept on a wooden bench.

Da Nang was a coastal city in the central part of the country and was the midway stop of my journey north to Quang Tri. It had beautiful sandy beaches and was for a time a French colonial port. I thought that in the future it would become a modern tourist attraction. During the war it became a target during the Tet Offensive. I did come back here during the latter part of my tour to visit its wonderful beaches and enjoy its geography before moving on to my next assignment in Cam Ranh Bay.

After two nights in Da Nang, I finally made it to my final destination in Quang Tri in mid-November 1970. I arrived late in the day to report at my new position and to meet my medics and other officers. The evening I arrived was dark, cool, damp, and rainy. The temperature that early November was in the high forties—much cooler than I would have ever imagined. What a drab, depressing place. This was malaria country, and I had decided *not* to take my prophylactic medicine, chloroquine, because of fear of commonly known side effects like nausea, abdominal cramps, and diarrhea. The pills were made to be taken weekly.

My first evening in my new home environment was pleasant. I was tired, cold, anxious, and a bit scared—I could have been on another planet with an alien race. The men and other officers seemed friendly, engaging, and accepting of someone new and clueless. This was all new to me: a foreign place, military lingo, war, monsoon rain, mosquitoes, malaria, no flush toilets. We ate together, and I decided to take my first malaria prevention pill. I was now settled in and no longer traveling, so I thought it safe to start my medication. I was ready for any adverse gastrointestinal issues from these medications. It was now around 7:00 p.m.

Life is always interesting with twists and challenges. Everything can seem so right and comforting even when it's not. Within an hour or so after I had eaten with my new unit, there came an alert. Word was that we might be attacked by Viet Cong or whoever! We were under lockdown. No one was to leave any building. Hunker down. I had been here maybe three hours, and we were under possible attack! Are you fucking kidding me?! I had taken my pill in a time of calm and peace. Darkness and rain outside. Darkness and quiet inside. Nothing. All quiet, except the rain and my growling stomach, which began increasingly to cramp. Holy shit! This could not be good. The chloroquine was starting to bother my GI tract, and I was holed up with people I'd just met and couldn't leave to find a latrine. Wait it out? Could I wait it out? Options did not appear good if these cramps continued to get worse. Still dark and quiet. It was becoming obvious I needed to make a decision—either I was going to have an embarrassing event here among all these men I had just met, or I needed to find a latrine—a bathroom, a toilet! So I asked, "Where *is* the nearest latrine?"

They said, "You cannot leave—we're under an alert. If you're sneaking out and about outside in the dark and rain, someone can shoot at you!" At this point, I didn't care. I was going out—and I did! I had no idea where I was or where I was headed in the dark and rain, but I wasn't staying there. It was black outside, muddy, and quiet. I don't remember much about working my way through the dark and rain and mud and panic of that evening. All I can recall is that at some point—with great glee—I found the latrine, and I was not shot at by any side. I know I stayed in that latrine until daylight, and I went to work the next day—my first working day as the battalion surgeon of the First/Fifth Infantry. This was going to be a fun year!

There would be 365 days of an altered life. I had some consolation in knowing I had a date to leave—November 4, 1971. In the last big war, you fought until it was over. Now it was one year—get used to it. There was no place to hide. I thought, Don't show any fear or helplessness, no matter how much terror or sense of loss you hold. Always act as if you're in control of the situation—even if you are not. War brings your own vulnerability right to your front doorstep—when you see death and tragedy, you could be next. You mark the days and weeks, then the seasons. This accounting of passing time created a different problem I had not thought about. As time passed and the days remaining become scanty, there was a fraternity of short-timers—those whose numbered days were less than one hundred—and they felt they should be respected as having done their time. Now, let the new arrivals take the risks and go out into the bush to fight this stupid war. The sick call was filled with short-timers anxious not to die with only a few days left there. When do you define a short-timer? I asked myself.

What was there to dislike about Vietnam for me? Well, I was away from those I loved. Already while I was here, close relatives had died that I couldn't see. The food could've been better. My oncology training was on hold—I was fearful I was losing those gifts I'd worked so hard for the last two years. I was working at an aid station, caring for generally healthy young men—men who wanted any reason not to fight. I had no training, no equipment, no means to care for trauma. I was a sanitation officer—keeping toilets going. These were healthy, scared men, unless shot or blown up. However, the weather sucked—hot, humid, and rainy during the monsoon season. Mud all around us. No flush toilets. Then there was the threat of malaria, malaria pills, rats, friendly fire, heroin abuse, helicopter crashes, venereal diseases, occasional shooting of officers by a disgruntled soldier, suicide attempts, alcoholism, and just plain going nuts here. We counted the days. Sometimes the men would take it out on a fellow soldier. Once they severely beat up someone who had hired a prostitute that spread a venereal disease—they broke his collar with a large piece of wood. We counted the days. I observed.

Was I afraid? I was uneasy about the possibility of dying—less about dying and more about dying there, in such a foreign place, lost forever to all those who loved me. I was twenty-eight years old when I arrived in Vietnam. Not that I was fearless, and I was certainly no hero type, but I found myself caught in the reality of my situation, which couldn't change, and I had no control over the situation. What bothered me more was my sense of the military's indifference if I perished there. I would be a possible casualty of the situation, another number among the numbers already counted. I didn't want to be part of that indifference, especially if my body could not be found—missing in action. I wanted to be grieved over and remembered by my family. At the time, I had no children—no legacy to leave. People would move on, but let them move on with my remains close. The dead, I realized, do matter, and that's why our burial rituals give meaning to the life lived. I wanted to be home. Would they even know I was dead, or worse, would my body be left behind here? I wanted to be grieved at home. And then one day rolled into another. We were not able to call home; there was no internet! Newspapers and letters came weeks later. News was always old.

I felt connected to the night sky. I was seeing the same sky, the same moon and stars—always a day ahead. I gave up trying to imagine or calculate the exact time of what possibly could be happening at home. I knew I was far from home. One adapts. One can be afraid sometimes—however, one cannot live this way all the time. You begin to trust those among you to somehow care for and protect you—and you them. We were all in this together—how I hate the phrase—but we were all together, wanting collectively to somehow get through this and get home.

I understand it now—the talk about army buddies. How intense and important these relationships with fellow soldiers became was striking to me. Yet I knew that when this year was over, this bonding would be no more—not after my 365 days. I felt real grief and future loss over this intense interconnectedness of people, all with the same purpose—getting home. I still, to this day, mourn the permanent loss of friendships that were born out of mutual trust, need, and purpose. If there is anything real and genuine about admitting I'm glad I served and was there, it is in having had the gift of profound comradery.

Christmas Day 1970 had been quiet. We finished our holiday turkey meal on the firebase in Mai Loc—a dug-out dirt mound supported to withstand mortar shells. We were reasonably comfortable inside, except for the large rats who roamed around nightly in the dark—occasionally nibbling at our feet in bed. The natives would catch and eat these rodents. I hated rats. We had been there for several days when I, out of boredom, constructed a picnic table from empty ammunition boxes that we kept on top of the mound. A few days before, we had treated a solder with massive doses of penicillin—I was convinced he had acute appendicitis, but because of bad weather conditions, we could not evacuate him. He did not make it out of the base—and he lived.

This Christmas Day had started sunny, but by midafternoon, wind and heavy rain moved in and changed the mood of the day. There had been an announced holiday cease-fire, which was common for that time. Not this Christmas. The lieutenant colonel was looking for me late in the afternoon. One of our soldiers out in the bush had been shot!

"How badly is he hurt?"

"Don't know."

"Where, exactly, is he?"

"Not sure."

"How am I going to help? I'm not a trauma surgeon, nor do I have anything to treat wounds."

"We're going to find him" was the order.

"I'm coming!"

The wind, rain, and increasing darkness now were formidable obstacles, at least to me. There was no way I was talking my CO out of taking me on a helicopter to find this wounded soldier. I didn't want to die on Christmas this way.

This was not the time to panic or think about possible negative consequences. I thought, Remember your own advice—don't ever show fear or helplessness. You can feel it, but don't show it! What could happen? Well, we were flying in a battle zone—I could be shot! The helicopter could crash or be shot out of the sky, and we would be lost in the jungle! We might not find him. He might be dead already. We flew at treetop level, swerving left, then right, to avoid being hit by gunfire. The wind and rain were worse. There was noise all about—the helicopter itself, the pounding rain, and the wind sounding off the vegetation. Now, we were out a good while—twenty or thirty minutes? There was to be a sign—a color drop locating the pickup spot of the injured soldier. Nothing. Still more noise. Now it was darker.

Finally, we saw the orange smoke pattern in the rain and gusty chaos and flurry of movement. Dear God, please no shooting! No explosions! We had to move - jump off the helicopter and move him quickly onto the bird hovering above. Noise! No gunfire. We were safely off the ground. Now to see how badly he was hurt. He was unconscious, cool, with weak but palpable pulses. Blood everywhere. There was a wound on the right side of the abdomen—I thought he had been shot in the liver. It didn't take long to realize the gravity of his situation. I forgot about the noise and the weather conditions and our predicament. I was a physician with certain skills; all was not lost. He was going to die unless we acted quickly and got him back to Quang Tri—to the main surgical hospital. How much time would it take to fly there? Could take close to an hour. I gave my recommendation. They listened. And we made the journey back to the brigade headquarters of Quang Tri. He survived surgery at Quang Tri, only to die later after his transfer to Japan.

It was months later when I met with my CO to talk about this man who had died after that Christmas attack. I wrote to his family about what I knew and had experienced that day. I was deeply saddened and sorry for their loss and wished I could have done more. I had witnessed the truth of war—the senselessness of loss—and I saw little glory or meaning here to celebrate. Was this the death of a hero, or did we make him a hero to give his death meaning and sanity? Of what value was this one death? I had seen death once again. My own life had been spared that noisy, windy afternoon. My family had been given a pass on the enormous loss that came home to that soldier's family that year. What a Christmas to remember! Grief would knock at their door.

There was a great deal of downtime in 'Nam—when I was not in the firebase or part of an invasion like the one into

Laos in February 1971, I can't say I worked hard. I took sick calls daily, seeing as few as twenty to thirty or as many as sixty to seventy young soldiers with a variety of minor ailments—usually related to the humid environs, to sexual misadventures usually on R and R in Thailand or Australia, or rarely to picking up something exotic like subacute bacterial endocarditis related to the dirty needles used for injecting heroin.

The medical aid station was two hundred feet away from where I slept—always in view. Screened walls and layered metal roofs made the heavy rain interesting—certainly noisy. Other living quarters were close, so you were condemned to the smells and music of the day. I remember working and hearing, for literally my entire five-to-six-hour aid station shift, loudly, the Bee Gees' "I Started a Joke" over and over and over. The area was reasonably safe from attack, although the Viet Cong had blown up our ammunition depot one night—quite a Fourth of July–like event. The worry was whether this was the start of a broader attack—and we did take it seriously. I missed learning. I missed having other physicians around. I missed reading about difficult cases. I missed feeling like a real doctor. I was something of a lost figurehead—most of the real medicine was at the main hospital with real specialists in Quang Tri or at the MASH units where helicopters brought the wounded.

Near the close of my tour in Quang Tri, in the springtime of 1971, something happened that gave me confidence again to be the good doctor. Things had quieted down after Khe Sanh, and our unit was starting to stand down. I was awaiting new orders, as I knew I was staying in 'Nam until November. The weather was improved—the monsoon season had ended. We were back at the safer large base at Quang Tri. Each night soldiers would set up mines to protect against the invasion of the Viet Cong enemy soldiers over the perimeter. They also would have helicopters shoot these "fishhooks" randomly at the outside of the base just in case the enemy was hidden, sneaking about. I was unaware of this practice at the time.

As Good As It Gets

The day was late but not dark. I remember it being sunny and warm. The showers were close to my modest residence, and I was washing up when I could hear my medics calling my name. Something had happened. One of the men who was setting up a mine might have been shot by friendly fire from the helicopter. I got dressed and within a brief time had ridden in our Red Cross jeep to the other side of the base. The soldier was still there on the ground. We arrived within ten minutes. He was alert and responsive, but clammy and short of breath. There was a small puncture wound, but not much blood or evidence of bleeding. Now he was coughing but not spitting up blood. My exam needed to be quick. The chest wall was flat—like when you're trying to find a wall stud to hang a picture. It meant there was no air moving in that lung. He had signs of fluid or blood in his lung.. I thought he was bleeding into the lung. We needed to get him to the main hospital on base quickly—now! I was again a physician, at least for today. He was saved by a good thoracic surgeon at the hospital. One of those needle fishhooks had punctured the thoracic aorta. I had helped beat and stall grief for another day. Hopefully, grief would delay its arrival in his family for many years to come—and I hope he lived a good life.

There are other memories of Vietnam that still haunt me. Things that bother the soul. My job as a battalion surgeon was to keep the soldiers healthy to go out and fight. Some had real issues that kept them back at the base camp, preventing them from having to go out on patrol in the bush. For grunts who were the short-timers with expected dates of departure less than one hundred days away, this feat became more difficult. The short-timers thought, Let new arrivals go out into the bush and get shot. I've paid my Vietnam dues. A particular private wanted out just for that very reason. No medical condition. No psychiatric diagnosis. He had the expected fear and anxiety any one of us would have in a war zone. There was no reason, as I recall, to give him a pass. He had come to me before with similar fears about his time in Vietnam. He was killed that next outing. One lives. One observes. One regrets.

Once at Khe Sanh, a helicopter landed near my Red Cross aid station and gave me a dead GI recently killed, probably shot. What the hell was I to do with a dead body? There were pictures in his uniform , probably his wife and kids. A name was on his tags. We loaded the body onto my Red Cross jeep and ventured to a MASH unit. Too much red tape—they didn't want the corpse. I asked what they wanted me to do with him. Shouts of "Bury the poor bastard!" came back—God, no way. I didn't want to end up dead there, left behind, forgotten. No fucking way! The MASH unit did take him, and I assume his body got back home—but I really don't know.

I was in charge of "public health"—I watched for any signs of unusual illness, and I had control of waste management. As mentioned before, there were no flush toilets. Barrels would be used and filled with flammable stuff and burned. Did you know that shit burns? I didn't. The awe and majesty of the sight of shit barrels burning are beyond description or comprehension. From a great distance, one could witness the intense black smoke and flames coming from the half-cut barrels, and by this sign one could identify a civilization of soldiers, and I was in charge of this endeavor. I built the latrines and decided where they ended up, and I was proudly in control of the waste management. The shitters stood out, scattered about the "campus" of the base. The flames burned a long time, reducing the feces to respectable ash, so fuel needed to be added in just the right proportions. When we moved into Khe Sanh in February 1971, the time of the Lam Son 719 operation to support South Vietnamese troops, several hundred of us arrived in this hell of a place the marines had fought in years before—sand, dry emptiness. Hot, dry, empty land. We did not carry mobile toilets but needed to build them with the empty wood cartons that had carried ammunition. There was a brief disagreement about where each latrine would go—everybody wanted one close by. As commander of latrines, I had to find answers. I screamed, "We'll build shitters everywhere! I'll cover the landscape with them! A latrine per man if you want!"

Then there was a controversy because my men had cut square toilet seats. You really couldn't satisfy anybody. Shitting became a new experience over square seats. There was an element of adventure we created with each new latrine, even with a door you could close for privacy, and close to your foxhole to boot. Soldiers would write poetic notes on the wooden walls of the latrines—such wit and wisdom. "Fighting for peace is like fucking for chastity." "You know why Colonel Townes never unloads his gun? He doesn't know how to load it." "Lifers are like flies—they eat shit and bother people." I really wanted to go home.

I think what made it somewhat bearable for me was the fact that my father and his three brothers, my uncles Louie, Frankie and Robbie, had all served in World War II. They didn't have a one-year tour and then return home—they had to endure until it was over. I thought a lot of my dad. He was destined to invade Japan from Okinawa.

Seven months before I came to Vietnam, my father and I went to the wake of his cousin's son- young soldier. He had been hit by a mortar shell and died instantly. He was the only child of my father's cousin. It ended her marriage and, I suspect, her life as she knew it. At the wake, my father and I stood as she sobbed and screamed at me not to go. She begged me to escape over the Canadian border. I thought how incredibly difficult this must have been for my dad—torn with the concern and fear that any father with a child going off to war would have. But he had done it. No words were ever spoken to me by my father about that day. Nothing was said to my mother about that terrible scene at the wake. I never really ever considered not going—I had hoped, like many at the time, that the war would end soon. One always thinks the best when one is afraid, and I did exactly that—How bad can this be? I learned that lesson.

Our military operation in February 1971 into Khe Sanh taught me better about the army, about the connection of comradery I had always heard about, and about fear for my life. Our mission was this: my infantry unit was to guard the airstrip where planes landed in support of the South Vietnamese, who were to invade Laos with our air assistance. It took us eight to nine hours to get there during the night from Quang Tri in a long military caravan. They told us to go around 11:00 p.m. I wasn't allowed to drive, so I sat up front—go and stop all night. The weather was hot, but at least there wasn't rain. I heard and saw no rockets and heard no gunfire. I had no idea why or where we were going except Khe Sanh. No one gave me any heads-up about what my job was or how dangerous this was. I had a backpack. I had my .45-caliber pistol (which I never cleaned or used).

By sunrise, we had reached a flat, treeless, dry area—miles of just nothing, with small distant hills. The weather was warm, the morning somewhat more comfortable. We sat in the jeep and waited and waited and waited. Finally, in the late morning, almost noon, we moved into the terrain we were to settle. This was on a hill overlooking the obvious airstrip they had talked about. This would be home for the next sixty to ninety days. We set up our red-crossed tent as an aid station and were told to start digging underground foxholes to prepare for the expected mortar fire to come. And we dug and dug and dug until we had a hole deep in the ground where four of us could sleep. We covered the hole with metal sheets and then layer upon layer of sandbags that we filled. I was in the best shape of my life—no doctoring, but I could dig large holes.

It came to me that we would be sleeping in the dirt with insects and rats, and who knows what atrocious animals could be there around us. I had a clever idea to take our stretchers—we never used them—place rope around the stretcher handles, and loop the rope over the roof we'd constructed. We'd sleep on the hanging stretchers—we would be at least free of the mud, bugs, and water when it rained. Occasionally the wall would blossom with thousands of larvae—but we got immune to this annoyance. We were nearly settled when the mortar rockets finally showed up—usually 6:00 to 7:00 a.m. and at dusk. Pretty much on schedule. We would count them as they whistled over us and exploded. The highest count was eighty, and there was only one death.

The threat of the enemy trying to kill us was always unsettling. The Viet Cong and North Vietnamese were trying to kill me! We would huddle under the sandbags and await the end of a seemingly endless number of rounds overhead. You felt good when you could hear the screeching sound—it usually meant the rounds would explode away from you. Occasionally, you would get caught outside and hopefully not in a latrine. And then it would end—the quiet returned, and you would move about again. Even this we could adapt to.

The night the South Vietnamese entered Laos was finally upon us. The operation was called Lam Son 719 and was designed to hinder construction of the Ho Chi Minh Trail, the main supply route for the North Vietnamese Army. We were told that none of our troops were to be involved. I don't recall details of the day, but I remember being called upon to go to the MASH unit not too distant from where we were based. This was where injuries were treated, where helicopters dropped off the wounded. Why was I needed? Why the urgency? There were no more than five or six physicians there when I reached the MASH tent. We were expecting many casualties in the next hour—all South Vietnamese soldiers. The word was that our planes had accidentally dropped bombs on the "good guys." The night was nasty. The wind began to pick up, and heavy rain and some fog added to the impending onslaught to face us. What was my role? What the hell did they want me to do? Someone needed to triage the incoming—separate out the salvageable from those deemed doomed. Not something I'd learned in medical school or in internal medicine residency training. I don't remember fear—just anxious anticipation of what I would see. We quickly got acquainted with the layout and with each other.

Then, in the distance, we could hear the unforgettable buzzing of multiple birds getting louder and louder. They were coming. Unmistakable noise. Now there was wind from the weather and the birds. Suddenly, it was here—organized, fretful chaos, one casualty after another after another. I had never seen, and never have since, such slaughter and blood and ripped-off extremities, or more blood and pain and moaning and death. Everything occurred in a blurred, cloudy reality—it happened, and I acted, did what needed doing and moved on with time for later reflection. No space for questioning—is this OK or not OK? No, this is what I'm doing—follow my orders and my lead. Get the potential living to where they can be treated. Let the dead be placed with the dead. And somehow the night ended, and people went back to where they had started—no overview or postmortem of what had just happened. Put this away—observe and hopefully go home.

After this rousing experience, things around the base seemed to quiet down. We were headed back to Quang Tri soon. There were fewer of us around. It felt as if there were too few of us around, and why wasn't I going back with these troops? The chaplain was back. I had little to really offer, but I was a physician—it made people feel better if a real doctor, not just a medic, was here with them. There was even a threat that the Viet Cong could attack—that we were vulnerable and had better stay up, take turns standing watch, just in case. Pray for a full moon—nobody was crazy enough to attack at a full moon. I had my medic clean my .45-caliber pistol, and I took a few hours to stay up and watch. Were they fucking kidding me? I had never fired this weapon. We didn't think about going out to pee—it was dark, quiet, and nobody was sure what was going on. We were given no orders or instructions—we just waited.

We began to move out from the Khe Sanh base that had been home the last two months. We walked and walked some more. Where the hell were we going now? By the third evening, we were getting nervous—we no longer had the protection of foxholes, sandbags, and numbers. Our Vietnamese scout told us he was concerned—he warned us that if we stayed here in this place one more night, the North Vietnamese would have us in their sights. Sure as shit, it was dusk, quiet—suddenly, no whistle, just a loud explosion fifty feet to my left. Holy shit! Mortar fire. We hit the earth, and I buried myself as close as I could. Another blast, and a third. I could feel warm shrapnel on my back—no pain and no injury, but the explosions were scaring the shit out of me. There were maybe two to three more shells fired at us, and it was over. That was the last time I ever was fired upon again in 'Nam. None of us were injured, just somewhat nervous it could start again, but it never did. And then—like every other time—we ate and fell asleep hoping tomorrow the bastards would pick us up.

We found a beautiful river and multiple waterfalls the next afternoon. No one had bathed for weeks. I felt seedy. There may have been a couple hundred of us—we threw our clothes off and jumped into this beautiful paradise of a place. The noise of the water falling was life giving—cool, fresh, clean water. There was a small incline, a ledge, where I took my camera and began to snap photographs of naked GIs trying to baptize themselves collectively. What joy those moments were—until we heard gunshots. Shit—they got us vulnerable and naked. We ran and got under cover—again, it was all over. We got word that the helicopters were on their way. We were to get picked up in the field. One after another they arrived—the welcomed birds we had waited for. We were going home to the home base at Quang Tri. But one of the soldiers was killed that day. A picture I took of him hangs in my home office, a reminder that we were not in the Garden of Eden, at least not before the fall of man. I had lived through shit—I wasn't really sure how or if I was better for this experience. But I observed.

The war was winding down. Our unit, the First/Fifth Infantry unit, was standing down and going home, but not me. I didn't have enough days in 'Nam to return with the unit. What hellhole awaited me next? I was still no more credentialed than before, so I was mildly nervous about where to, but I ended up at Cam Ranh Bay, specifically the drug detoxification center. This was a good thing. Safe and a medical mission, albeit related to drugs. What was happening at that time was that young GIs were easily getting addicted to heroin, which was cheap and available. The long plane ride home had reported many episodes of opioid withdrawal—not a pretty picture. The base "hospital" drug detoxification was in a safe, enviable place. To the east was the South China Sea. Small islands coated the landscape, with picturesque small fishing boats scattered about. No threat there. To the west, a short distance away, was the US Air Force base from which, in November 1971 I would leave to go home. All I needed was a jeep ride. To the north were South Korean troops—tough and in place. I would be one of a dozen or more captain physicians who would admit those poor bastards who were getting on a "big bird" home but who had tested positive for narcotics in their urine. So imagine! I was to admit fifty to sixty guys who had just spent a year here in 'Nam—mostly against their will, in an unpopular war—and tell them, "Can't go home!"

I worked one out of every fourteen to fifteen nights taking care of new arrivals to the drug detoxification center. This was not a bad deal. We were right on the South China Sea on a gorgeous sandy beach, albeit one with barbed wire. The water was warm, and the view of small islands across the bay was spectacular, especially at night, when the fishermen were out in small lit boats. However, the nights that I was on duty were usually tense. The men recently taken from their rides home after a year in Vietnam were noisy, rowdy, and angry. I was supposed to do a quick physical exam, process them into the hospital, and get them into their beds, which indeed were in a prison, with gates and military police guarding the place. There were occasional riots with buildings set ablaze, but I never felt too threatened. Remember, I had been in Vietnam nearly a year by this time. Little could fluster me now.

The nights we got these new admissions were hot and sticky. We were all irritable. We got as many as eighty new admissions to the camp on a good night. I remember once when there were two of us on duty to handle the large load of retained soldiers. It was a particularly hot and humid evening. Things were moving slowly, and everyone was becoming more irritable and agitated. We requested that the administrator in charge, a nurse with the rank of major, help get us an air conditioner. No help there. More tension grew, as it was obvious this was to be a long night. My doctor partner and I said no. We would not see another admission until we got relief in the form of a cold-producing machine. We didn't care if they burned the place to the ground! In any case, where it came from, I do not know, but we had an air conditioner for the small examining area, and the night ended like all others. I love the army.

During the daytime, we would round and check on the patients clinically, making sure no one was going into opioid withdrawal, and we also monitored any levels of opioids left in their blood. If all was well, they were discharged, usually after a three- or four-day stay. They were placed back on the big bird home. Occasionally, there was a serious event. For example, in examining one soldier, we saw signs of endocarditis, a serious infection of the heart valves with staphylococcus. This can be a deadly illness related to intravenous drug abuse and must be treated quickly and correctly with antibiotics. He was transferred back to a military hospital. We kept no outcome records of our hospital's clientele, and I do not know if the army followed up on all these individuals over time.

The patients would need to stay until there were no signs of opioid dependency or withdrawal symptoms. They did not take this well. All of us were captains except two majors and the commander, who was a colonel. As it turned out, I was the highest-ranking captain—turned out this became important.

Sometime in late September or October 1971, I was called to the headquarters office. I wondered what I had done. The colonel was going to Japan on R and R to meet his wife. The two majors also would be on some type of leave. The drug center required a physician to be in charge. That person was me.

"Are you kidding about this?" I asked.
"No," was the response.
"How long a period of time?"
"Maybe two weeks."
"Are you kidding me?"

"No."

A new adventure for me. Could I close the place? No. I was to make sure the medical operation remained professional and ensure the right personnel did their jobs. And by the way, there was an important Pacific general coming to make an inspection.

"Are you kidding me?"

"No."

I wanted more than ever to be home and not here. When I arrived for my first morning of work, the administrator, a lieutenant colonel, asked me to take the commander's office seat. I declined and suggested that he outranked me by two ranks, so he should sit there in the impressive chair. He insisted this is where I was to sit. I gave in and sat. It was a comfortable, large chair. If you asked me now what I did those two weeks, I couldn't tell you. The general came, and I guess we passed, and I wasn't ordered to jail or even better, shot. It seemed quite a superficial examination, the questions not terribly probing. But what do I know? Then came the typhoon! That took work, energy, and my best organizational skills to keep us literally afloat. I was impressed with the rapid severe change in Mother Nature. I was upset the storm couldn't have waited at least a few days. It passed, the days moved by, and the colonel returned. The command personnel were nice. As the army does, they gathered a number of people and formed a ceremonial line, and I received a commendation medal that they added to my uniform. I would have preferred that they send me home.

Why do some people we meet stay with us for life? What is so special about these individuals that they remain in our memories, haunting us, even if that time spent with them was brief? Is it because the time we connect in is one where we are vulnerable and not in control? Often, this idea is seen in reverse: we see a pivotal point in our lives, a crossroad where we can go one way or take a totally different path. It was my last three months of my tour in Vietnam. I still had another year to serve in Virginia at Fort Eustis, and then I would go back to

As Good As It Gets

New York to start my oncology fellowship at Memorial Sloan Kettering Cancer Center. At the time I had been married the past five years without children, separated from my wife for most of that time because of medical school obligations, internship and residency time commitments, and now the war in Vietnam. I had married hurriedly at age twenty-three, much too young to appreciate the burden and longevity of married life. I was to head back home in early November 1971, and there was no doubt about that. The days that I was counting down seemed to be going too quickly and strangely. I wanted time to slow down. It was becoming a burden to think about returning to the States. How strange was this?

I was in the clinic office when I first met Beverly. She was in her twenties, blond, petite, with an infectious smile and good posture. She had a quiet poise and dignified calmness about her and asked if she could talk with me about a personal medical issue. She was told by the other nurses and women that I could be trusted and seemed to be a good doctor. I was, of course, flattered, and we fixed whatever it was that needed attention. I can't recall what the problem was. We spoke for a while and became good friends.

Bev was easy to like and talk to seemingly about everything. She was well read, raised in Milwaukee, Wisconsin. We spoke for hours about her life and plans, about my hopes and fears, and about our dreams for a better tomorrow. The war was a major topic, and by this time, I had a lot of stories and opinions.

My marriage had been flat, but at the time, it felt like the weather—I was not going to change it. I had future plans, and stupidly, I saw my marriage as a side part of my life, not as crucial as becoming a doctor or specialist. There was no life in this partnership, but at the time, I did not have enough energy to kill it. It was what it was. We were intimate strangers, and I began to dislike the thought of leaving this paradise for home. This was an awful, foreign, strange feeling for me. I would miss this place, these people I'd come to like and respect. The war had created a situation of forced, intense relationships that bound you to a place and time. Were they so intense because they were so fragile and time limited with an expiration date? I would miss all of it!

Beverly and I never spoke of our relationship as more than just one between good friends. A "we" was never established. No holding or kissing occurred; no words of romance were ever spoken. The innocence of it all, I believe, has kept the permanence of longing. It would be wonderful to think we could speak as in 1971 again, as two young people looking to the future. That train has long passed the station. The disappointment would be too hard to bear, and the yearning for something may be just better. We both knew that when I left, we would never see each other again. Why am I upset that she can remain only part of my past, a part that was brief and is now so vague? We're talking fifty years ago, and I would still like to say something.

When I was leaving to fly home, I went to say goodbye to Bev in her trailer. She was alone. I don't remember what I said except that I would miss seeing her. I kissed her on the forehead, gave her a bear hug, turned, and left. She gave me a card and said not to open it until the plane took off. The card had written quotes from Dag Hammarskjold's *Markings*. She wrote several quotes that reminded her of me. One read, "Every deed and every relationship is surrounded by an atmosphere of silence. Friendship needs no words—it is a solitude delivered from the anguish of loneliness."

I flew home on Flying Tigers Airlines. Soon after I read her card, we began to taxi, and then a loud bang announced that a tire had blown. We waited on the plane as they changed the tire. We took off, and then all the lights went out for a time. This was to be a memorable flight home. I was informed I was the highest-ranking officer on the plane if needed. I cried.

I can only wonder what the outcome of my life would have been if I had been there longer or decided to stay. What if I had sought romance and a new life? Was it a more meaningful relationship because it had to end? Some things need to die their natural deaths, and this relationship was one of them. I was to see death and grief in a different way. I suspect this has happened to soldiers in foreign places for a long time. I shouldn't think I was so unique. I admit to my vulnerability, but I also must confess that even after fifty-plus years, it still creates a sense of longing and wonder for me. Years later, my marriage did ultimately fail, and I did look back at a time long ago when someone briefly gave me the joy of living, and I knew what it was like and could try to find it again. I had done the right thing. I've never seen Beverly Ford again.

Ultimately, I did get home three days earlier than I was due—mainly because I had done some favor for some sergeant. And sergeants could do anything if they were in just that pivotal spot. I was quarantined behind barbed wire, got debriefed, had my urine checked for narcotics, and handed back my pistol with reluctance—we had become attached. I had said goodbye to my fellow physicians—they would soon follow. We all knew we would not see one another again. This was all for remembrance only. This intense bond would necessarily be broken—we would go our separate ways, so to speak. It was geography, life commitments, our responsibilities and duties to family and other people. This was a one-time false world—it was time to go home to the real world we all knew and wanted. Go home to those who knew us outside this insanity. The place in Cam Ranh Bay had actually been fun, and I could have seen myself staying there longer—if they had only asked. When I was promoted (purely a time thing) to major, I never purchased a major cap (for $100), which caused issues because a soldier couldn't be outside without a hat. Thus, I had to be driven everywhere back on the US base, Fort Eustis, in Virginia, where they sent me next.

We flew to Tacoma, Washington, that early November 1971—I would be home for the upcoming holidays. I kissed the ground when I got off the plane close to 9:00 or 10:00 p.m. that wonderful day. They kept us in a room for nearly two hours to give us news about home, fashion, music, and generally what was going on. I felt good, relieved to be on safe soil again—to feel safe among my people, though not quite whole.

A certain unfamiliarity stood within me, a jitteriness—I was not totally myself. The closeness of lots of people bothered me like I didn't remember. Sudden loud sounds startled me more than I could understand. I became more frightened when I reached New York City, a city I was accustomed to—Christ, I was born here; I used to thrive on crowds. This was a new feeling—a gift of Vietnam and war. But I was home, and I could hold my mother and make my father proud—I had done what he would have done for himself, and I knew he was happy I had paid the dues. I was tired of the pain and suffering I had witnessed—of children missing limbs, of soldiers crying not to go out in the bush, of taking orders in an exotic world that made no sense to me. I didn't want to think or talk about it, and I understood better why past soldiers kept silent about their time in the war. I was no hero. I hadn't done anything special or heroic. I showed up and was too scared to make a fuss or disrespect my father. Inside, I gave myself a pat on the back, and that was all that mattered.

The experience of war places a permanent stain on understanding human behavior and humanity itself. One reviews one's life with learned lessons, mostly about oneself—how one behaved in this test of character in a school one didn't wish to be in. I had taught myself, as I had as an intern, never to act helpless even when I felt helpless. Don't behave like you're uncomfortable with the situation. I think this was a genetic gift from my father, confronting life stuff as if you can win. Assume you belong there—it not only is what it is, but it was also meant to be what it is. In other words, act like your cat.

This "gift" came in handy for a funeral mass at St. Patrick's Cathedral in New York. A major donor had died, and this special High Mass was dedicated to him—large choir, tenor soloist , multiple priests, high ranking in the hierarchy of things. I was invited as the medical director of the hospital where he was a prominent donor. The mass was to begin at 9:00 a.m. on a Monday in Manhattan. I got there much too early and decided I needed coffee. After several cups I was back to the cathedral before everything started. People were getting seated. There was now some organ music in the distance. I had to pee. No question I would not last the hour-plus High Mass.

I got an usher to direct me to where a bathroom would be in St. Patrick's. I went down some stairs to where the old former cardinals are laid to rest. It was quite impressive to see all these tombs without much fanfare. The music now was heard, and there were some voices singing as well. The show had begun. It was a maze down there. Where the hell were the steps? I was now lost in the basement cemetery of St. Patrick's. Finally, I saw a stairway upward. The music was louder and the voices of the choir stronger. I stepped out onto the busy altar—in the middle of the altar at the start of this solemn mass in this holy, somber place. Priests all around—and me now in the middle of the altar. I decided to act as if I belonged. I walked *slowly* across the altar, acknowledging with a head nod the clergy I knew. I knew they were asking, "What the hell is he doing here?" I told myself, Act as if you are one of them. Act naturally. The music continued. I crossed the altar field and sat down in my place. The cathedral was filled with people who hopefully thought I had some reason to be there. Maybe someone was ill. I would act like a cat on a mission. Interestingly, no one ever questioned me.

By 1987, nearly fifteen years after I'd come home from Vietnam, my life had changed. I had finished my medical oncology fellowship at Memorial Sloan Kettering, and had worked in an academic oncology practice alongside Rodger Winn, a former attending, from MSKCC (who later helped establish standard national cancer treatment guidelines). I had settled in as the medical director of the hospital I had worked at during the night when I was a medical resident before going to 'Nam. I was completing my master's thesis, writing, and starting a teaching clerkship for a PhD-track bioethicist from Georgetown University's Kennedy Center for Bioethics. Ed Pellegrino was getting an award with us, and before the event, we talked, and he noted he had no clinical opportunity for these students. I said we could do it in New York—all I needed was some dollars to find a place for them to sleep, get them food money, and develop a syllabus. With some help from our fundraising, we had it established—what fun to teach bright, enthusiastic young scholars of the art of medicine and real-time ethical questions. With added support from MSKCC and people I knew at Albert Einstein Medical School across the street—Ruth Mackin; Nancy Dubler, an attorney at Montefiore Hospital; Paul Armstrong, the attorney for Karen Ann Quinlan—we began a clinical ethics practicum.

I finally got my MA in philosophy from Fordham and was doing what I loved doing—seeing patients, helping form some research questions in palliative medicine, teaching bright, enthusiastic students, and writing what I considered to be thoughts of a death watcher and what I viewed as philosophical oncology. And by the way, this is where I first met my Jane, whom I would ultimately marry in June 1993. I was content and happy collaborating with good, smart local colleagues like Russell Portenoy, Jimmie Holland, and Bill Breitbart in New York, and with people as far away as Japan, such as Kunihiko Ishitani in Sapporo. I was asked to contribute a chapter titled "Specialized Care of the Dying" to the main oncology text by Vincent DaVita and others and all this allowed me to think out those questions that had been with me from the beginning. In 1999, this contribution would win an award for the best chapter on end of life care.

I remember Woody Allen's words regarding life—that most of it is about just showing up. I've given up on free will. I would not have predicted that I'd spend a lifetime with Jane, move to the South—Atlanta, and eventually Charleston, South Carolina—have six children, including an adopted Chinese daughter, work at Emory University School of Medicine and the Medical University of South Carolina, and grow older without Jane, but with a renewed sense of the importance of living, working, spending time with children, and—embarrassing to admit—seeking romance and enriched love. When I was thinking about becoming a physician and later an oncologist, I continually focused on the next steps in my life—where would I live and practice? My vision was way off from the reality that happened. Now I tend to think backward, looking at life in reverse, trying to retrace how the hell I got here—what decisions worked or didn't and how many regrets there were to plug into my life's equation. What have I learned about these questions, which have been shaped by my oncology profession, my life experience, and my existential anxiety? What are the thoughts of a death watcher?

Many years before we were married, Jane wanted me to face my Vietnam demons. There was a New York Vietnam remembrance peace parade on May 8, 1985. She spent the day there. I could not face my demons then. I had safely, after my one-year tour, returned home and completed my military service obligations in 1972 at Fort Eustis in Virginia. I had recurrent nightmares during those early homecoming years. Always the same—I was back in Vietnam, doing another tour. Loud and sudden explosions of noise would startle me. Indeed, the first weeks back in New York City seemed menacing—too many people, too much energy and movement, and much too many sounds. Often, I would wake in the night fearful of a noise or a dream. These fears have all been resolved. I would have to face grief and death again, but it would be different and more difficult.

PART V:
Jane—Reflections on Love and Loss, Grief, and Guilt

How does it all start—a life and a love story? What are the ingredients that compose a "good marriage," that make it sustainable and livable so the couple doesn't have to stay together out of spite or for the children? I love the tale of the ninety-five-year-old married couple seeking a divorce and the attorney asking, "Why now?" "We wanted to wait until the children died," was the reply. Or there's Groucho Marx's comment: "Beware the couple holding hands because if they let go, they'll kill each other."

I really am not sure what made this marriage, Jane + Frank, so intractably good. I had given up my singularity and joined a "we." We did this. We did that. It was always assumed I would die first and she and all her close friends would be sitting on rocking chairs remembering the past. My father had died a week into his sixtieth year—he had five brothers, all dead from cardiovascular disease or stroke. Except for the oldest, they had destructive lifestyles—my father was overweight, smoked two to three packs of Camels a day until his midforties, never exercised, and had hypertension to boot. He also had deadly genes, mainly from his mother's side of the family. Jane's mother had died of breast cancer at age sixty-two, totally rejecting any diagnostic help or treatment—presenting with brain metastasis as evidenced by Bell's palsy. Women whose mothers die of this seem to suffer more—from the anticipation that they will get breast cancer as well and then from the disease itself. Her poor father had to witness both his wife and daughter suffer the ravages of this disease. But we don't live by threats of dying of whatever future ailment—we live our lives just trying to survive the cost of living and the weather.

I watch my ninety-six-year-old and ninety-two-year-old in-laws, who have been married since the early 1950s. Long-lasting love has merged them as one—they are so dependent that I suspect when one goes, the other will soon follow. Love's true, long-standing connection like this makes the torment of grief so much more vivid and catastrophic, so we believe either in the nothingness of the dust believers and the contradiction of wasting so much effort to love, or in the idea that we'll meet again—but that demands real faith. As Robert Nozick writes in his wonderful little book *The Examined Life*, love's common bond causes an extension of our being—when a loved one suffers, we suffer. We live in this extension from within us—we are most satisfied, content, and happy even with ourselves. That someone could love me with all my faults is a wondrous thing. And if my father-and mother-in-law can stand each other for that long, that's love.

The uncertainty of meeting someone new is exciting—trying to go up the learning curve of another is both rewarding and frightening. It takes energy and sleepless nights and singing a new song—and then fifty-plus years go by, and there is love and accepted certitude about who the other person is. And we conclude, ultimately, that this love is good—that the partner chosen is the one, the only one we wish to stay with—to see first in the morning and last at dark. We think, I know this person, even in the biblical sense, and this person knows me. There is no need to trade up from a "Chevy" person to a "Mercedes" person—the positives outweigh the negatives.

It's wonderful to see love in my patients for their spouses, parents, and children, where death comes without guilt or greed but just as an expected grief, sorrow, and loss. Often, I'm surprised how deep the sacrifice goes to care for a loved one and all that implies—just changing and cleaning the dirty sheets on a bed can be a formidable and unrewarding task. At times I assumed the presence of love at the wrong times. I recall a patient who was in my care dying of advanced ovarian cancer—in pain, weak, hospitalized, and weeks away from death. Then her husband died suddenly. No children. No other close relatives. She needed to go and persuaded us to let her go to his burial—her words after the funeral were telling: "I had to see the son of a bitch in the ground." That will wake your senses, much more than Death Wish coffee. He had been an abusive man. She passed away as expected, but much later, with less pain. And I suspect much happier. I believe that if she could, she would have thrown worms on his grave site.

How did it all start for me? How did the two of us evolve from individuals to an ontological "we"—Jane and Frank? The first time I can remember seeing Jane was at a December 1983 hospital Christmas party—a large affair with several hundred people crammed into the ballroom of the Bronx Marina Del Rey on Long Island Sound. I was separated and alone. Jane showed up with a tall, dark, and handsome *GQ* guy. She had been hired by Patricia Cahill, who later headed the Catholic health system of the New York Catholic Archdiocese. Jane was recruited to help with human resource management at Calvary, where I had become the medical director three years before she was hired. This was the same place where I had moonlighted before Vietnam. She was to spiff up and improve the personnel department—help with time management, review policies relating to education and sexual harassment, and so forth. She was bright, attractive, full of life and laughter, animated, and, I assumed, married. She later told me that she thought I was interesting.

Not to bore you…we became good friends, went to lunch and dinner, but never dated—she was exceptional. I was nervous then about her. She was a dynamo—a bundle of talented energy. She left Calvary in 1985, went to Atlanta, started her own business, and married a childhood friend of her brother—a tall, good-looking, blond, a monotonously speaking lawyer or accountant. I quietly thought this could not last. I declined an invitation to the wedding—this was in 1987. Her marriage became rocky; marriage counselors were called. In May 1991, her car broke down while she was living in Columbia, South Carolina. "Miss Fix It" got out of the car, which was off to the side of the road, opened the hood, and had gone back to get in the car when a physician's wife on a car phone caught her between her oncoming Chevy Suburban and the front door. Jane had a massive pelvic fracture, internal bleeding, and a ruptured bladder and came close to death. Her friends phoned me to tell me the news—that she was critically ill and that she might never walk again. I called immediately and spoke to her in her hospital bed. She was obviously on narcotics—she had a slurred, slow, deliberate, weak voice. I asked if it was OK to call again, and I did.

In September, she was to be discharged to go home—her marriage was now truly over, as her husband wasn't aiming to handle a "cripple." Jane was told he had been having an affair while she was hospitalized. She told me the news about her situation and that she was planning a trip to New York to see about potential work. October was when I first saw her—frail, wasted, in pain, and in a wheelchair. We had tea at the Waldorf-Astoria at around four in the afternoon. I had not seen Jane for five years. She was in a bright green dress. I told her she reminded me of Kermit the Frog—a good pickup line! She asked what I thought about her moving to New York with help from a nanny for both herself and her one-and-a-half-year-old son, Matthew. The next February, she was in New York. Within three years, we were married. Almost ten years to the day after I met her—I would smile a lot. Almost twenty years to the day, she would be dead. I guess knowing her thirty years is what I should be grateful for. Suffice it to say I loved that she saw something in me that—pardon the triteness—made me more confident and self-aware of my salvageable qualities, helped me have a purposeful and decent life.

It was a June morning in 2004 when Jane asked me to just feel this area she had found on her left breast. A definite something was palpable—real enough that it needed attention. I had the luxury of just picking up the phone and calling a breast oncology surgeon, Paul Baron, that hour. By day's end, we knew this was breast cancer—within days we knew the type, the stage, and where treatment was going. I told Jane I would not interfere—would not "doctor"—but wanted to be a husband. I would interfere only if I strongly believed we should do something different than advised. And I kept my promise—and I have no guilt about how and where things went.

I was a breast medical oncologist, a professor, no less, with a long history of caring for dying people, facing death head on in my bedroom. Treatment decisions when she was initially diagnosed in 2004 had been made without delay. She had endured and paid her dues- including bilateral mastectomies, and systemic chemotherapy with the big guns—four cycles of Adriamycin and Cytoxan followed by Taxol. No radiation was indicated, and she underwent a brief trial of endocrine therapy with drugs like tamoxifen and later letrozole. She was fifty-three years old. She did not take chemotherapy well; she experienced nausea, vomiting, severe fatigue, and depression over her bodily losses—nothing I wasn't familiar with seeing. Yet I found language hard to talk through with her regarding what to expect or not expect—indeed, we are all so unique. She looked like a *Schindler's List* survivor in those early years of treatment, but it wasn't long before she was back in typical Jane form. Those who knew her recognized her tenacity, intelligence, curiosity about life, liberalism, kindness, and devoted loyalty. She was an uncomplaining, get-it-done kind of person. So damn smart! She had sailed in a forty-foot boat from Seattle to Hawaii, jumped out of airplanes, carried the

Olympic torch in Atlanta in 1996, been knighted at the Plaza Hotel (becoming Dame Jane), and married me! This was the only fault I could find with her—what was it about me? She had this infectious, hearty laugh that would bellow. She made best friends quickly, and all my male friends loved her more than they loved me.

We almost forgot the threat that was there—the risk for recurrence. We focused on the DSF—disease-free survival. And then in a moment seven and a half years later, in December 2011, she asked that I feel a bump on her arm. Suddenly, everything changed. Much worse than the original assault was this bump on her arm. Eighteen months later, my Jane was struggling to breathe her last—and she was laid to rest in our bed that Wednesday afternoon in June 2013. No more battle. Suffering and the sufferer were gone.

On December 14, 2011, she awoke quietly, as on any other morning. We had sold our house and decided to try renting a place in downtown Charleston, close to Colonial Lake. It was a nice and quiet neighborhood full of old homes with typical Charleston charm. After my shower, as I was ready to head for work, Jane asked me to feel something on her left forearm. Our adopted daughter, Joy, was on her way home from college for the Christmas break. I palpated the small mass she was feeling—I knew almost immediately that what I was feeling was not good—a recurrence, most likely, of her breast cancer that was initially diagnosed in 2004. I had little doubt. "Oh shit!" This was in my mind. Was this stage 4 disease and now incurable? Let's confirm, I thought.

I called Paul Baron, her breast surgeon, immediately from the bedroom. He would see her that morning. Seven and a half years had passed. She was feeling as well as ever. How could this happen? What had I done wrong? What had I missed doing? I didn't want her to have to do this again—everything, in a moment, had changed. All in life that's banal becomes meaningless. It was difficult during the first go-round in 2004—this was going to be more difficult. The likelihood, I thought, that this was the only area of disease was probably small—this might not be curable. One can begin to grieve too soon. I knew too much about this illness; more of a problem was that, knowing Jane, she would want to know and hear what I was thinking, what I *really* thought. That was who she was.

The biopsy proved the diagnosis to be recurrent breast cancer. The cancer was now biologically more aggressive, high grade, poorly differentiated, with the estrogen receptor remarkably lower, only 6 percent positive—an unfavorable sign. Her staging scans, however, were negative, meaning there was no gross, obvious evidence of metastatic disease in vital organs like the liver, lungs, or bones. The biopsy was positive, but it was taken from a lymph node, not skin—this was not stage IV disease. I suggested to Jane that we seek a second opinion at UNC-Chapel Hill with a breast medical oncologist, Dr. Lisa Carey. That led to genetic testing of the cancer in a clinical trial and total surgical left axillary lymph node dissection, followed back home with radiation. Now, we had no evidence of the remaining disease.

I was content with this current outcome—no evidence of disease (NED) and a sense of hope that the battle could be won. I raised the possibility of further limited adjunct chemotherapy, to Jane's disappointment and fear. I wanted Jane cured. In a quiet moment, Dr. Carey had Jane alone and said, "You know you don't have to do chemotherapy." Jane got the message early. She wanted the final surgical pathology report—there were forty-five positive cancer nodes removed! All these lymph nodes were poorly differentiated—a bad prognostic picture. Repeat staging scans remained clear, and for a brief time, there was some piece of mind, and we could think and talk about other things.

November 2012 approached—it was nearly a year to the date of her recurrent cancer biopsy. Per protocol, staging studies were again ordered by her treating local breast oncologist, Dr. Rita Kramer. She was on no treatment regimen but observation and surveillance. Jane felt well—did everything with her typical gusto. She didn't ask me any questions about what I thought or if I was nervous or concerned. I never examined her. I took the difficult road as the spouse. I did not seek to review her records or bring up conversation regarding her illness.

We had gone to New York that fall, as we often did—seeing several plays in a few days. She was up for it. The weather in New York was cold and damp. We were looking to get half-price play tickets at the Times Square TKTS booth. The holiday line for these coveted seats was formidable—it would be a long wait. At that time, they required cash only, and there was a huge, muscular, don't-fuck-with-me guy guarding the line and protecting it from being broken into. "Shit," I said. "Let's go. I don't want to wait in line—plus, it's too cold!"

I watched Jane survey the situation, looking at the line of people, then the guard, and back again at the line. She said, "I got it!" I thought, What has she got? Jane said, "I figured it out. Wait here." She removed cash from her purse and walked briskly toward the guard. "Sir, I went to get cash at the ATM machine over there. I was already in line, and they told me to come back for the tickets." No words from this guy. He gestured for her to go next. We had our tickets. That was my Jane. How well she looked.

When we got home to Charleston, the repeat staging scans were not good. I remembered coming home to find Jane sobbing quietly in our bedroom. The liver was showing metastatic lesions. Maybe something in the lung. I had nothing to say. There was nothing to say. We both knew the meaning of these results. She said she did not want to tell anyone—not her father, sister, or brothers, or the children. I wanted not to talk about it with any of them. I agreed not to say anything to anyone she didn't want to know.

By December 2012, I could begin to notice small but real differences in how she looked and moved—some weight loss, a little cough, and maybe some shortness of breath. Certainly, she got fatigued and needed more naps. Chemotherapy was again started, with the goal now not to cure her illness but to add more time. The bar of hope had been moved—not for more chemotherapy but for a more livable life. Side effects were always present and added to her already weakening state. I saw no improvement. Then the question from Jane: "What's my best estimate about time?" I was not surprised by the question coming from this no-nonsense woman. A surprisingly low number of my patients would come right out and ask it that way. Families would ask, but rarely my patients. I always portrayed a more reasonable optimistic number, never unrealistic. However, Jane was someone I loved deeply, and I became saddened by even imagining her gone from me. It alters your perception of prognostication. Christ, I was her husband, not her oncologist.

I realized quite soon that her question about remaining time was more about me than about her. She was preparing me for my life alone, without her around to care for me. She essentially said, "This is what you need to know—about insurance, bills, and taxes. This is where I keep all the papers, phone numbers, and names of people to call for help. Where should you live?" (We were renting in downtown Charleston.) "This is what you need to know about the kids' tuition and people at school to talk with, if necessary." She began visiting the homes, condominiums, and townhouses for sale. She, unknown to me at the time, would meet with very close friends- such as Judge Paul Garfinkel and his wife, Susan, saying, "Frank will need guidance! He probably shouldn't be alone after I'm gone." I would need much watching. I still, to this day, ten years after her death, find notes and hidden tips around the house for me about what I should or need to be doing.

In January of the year she died, we again went to New York. Chemotherapy was again to start, and again she would lose her hair. The indignity of it all. Macy's was giving up its wig salon, and there were sales. I tagged along to help choose one with her. She was feeling pretty good on that trip, as I recall. We had purchased an apartment in 2007 at the Metropolitan Towers on Fifty-Seventh Street, close to the Russian Tea Room near Seventh Avenue. We had rented it and had delusions that we could perhaps divide our time, when and if I retired, between Charleston and New York City.

The apartment was expensive to maintain, but we loved it. From the living room, you could see ice skaters in Central Park, and from the bedroom, you could see the Hudson River to the west and the East River to the east. Again, an example of Jane's intelligence: the apartment had been rented almost continually from the time we bought it. It was a great place—even the musical playwright Jerry Herman was interested in renting it when he needed a place in New York for a revival of *Mame*. That never happened, but it would have been fun if it had. He was ill, and someone else rented. The major storm Sandy hit the Northeast with a remarkable fury that season. Our renters had recently moved to find a larger place. The construction crane across Fifty-Seventh Street had become loose and crashed into our window on the fifty-fifth floor. No major damage, but the window needed to be fixed. The apartment was empty and not rented. Jane had added a waiver to the home insurance policy so that if something like this occurred, the company would have to give us full rent for six months! And the company honored the policy. We took the time that January to do some renovations of the kitchen and paint the place. We owned the apartment outright, but I think I slept there only three times. The apartment was in Jane's name, and she recognized what that could mean for me.

The time for her was closing in by May. On Mother's Day, again in New York with our adopted daughter, I remember her weeping at lunch when Joy left to go to the bathroom. She was timebound and knew the future was limited. How hard it is for us to be without tomorrows—all taken from us. The regret of what could have been and the sadness of not being among us. She was weaker, gaunt, with little appetite, and certainly more withdrawn. There was little laughter from her now. Her beloved first cousin, Bill Usinger, had died suddenly of a massive heart attack on Saint Patrick's Day that year. That May they would spread his ashes in the waters of Fort Lauderdale, where he grew up. Jane was invited to participate, along with his sisters, wife, and two children.

I asked her, "Do you really want to do this?" and she replied, "Yes." We decided—actually, I decided—to drive from South Carolina rather than fly. I wanted time—close, real, honest-to-goodness time to be able to talk with her. She did most of the driving, to my surprise, and felt well enough to maintain the trip. She did well.

Her cancer was progressing. There was no doubt. The chemotherapies were not showing any benefit. She was offered a phase 1 trial, the material for which she took to read on this road trip to Florida. She read the material, like only Jane could read something, while I drove. She put it down and asked me if I would be upset if she declined going on the trial. She was tired of fighting, tired of doctors, tired of blood sticks, and tired of hoping. It was too exhausting to hope anymore. I agreed with her. I really did. I was tired too! Hope can become an enemy, especially if you get off track and forget what you're hoping for, and it may be for the wrong thing—certainly not more chemotherapy and all it offers.

She helped scatter Bill's ashes. He was an engaging, smart, funny guy we had both loved to be with. He was always the right person to have a glass of wine with and talk to for hours about anything. I watched her as she walked into the beautiful, warm Atlantic waters, and I tried to imagine what she was thinking—about herself and tomorrows. I questioned whether coming to do this had been such a good idea, but when I asked her, she was adamant. "I need to do this." For whatever reason, she found peace here, and I thought maybe she felt a connection to Bill, one only she could know, and something more eternal in that ocean—something larger than herself. I don't know. I observed.

Those left behind have to bear the gift and the curse of last words. I still am haunted by Jane's: "I can't breathe! I can't breathe." I have to go further back: "It's not your fault—not your fault!" Words linger like bitterness or sweetness, not like a taste but like a mental hiccup. It would seem to me that the one dying is in the driver's seat—get it all out, tell the son of a bitch what you think, what you always thought. This seldom happens. There are always muddled questions left open, unanswered—I wondered what Jane *really* thought of me. Was I the idiot I thought I was? I wanted to clear up all the mysteries I'd never asked about us. Was I a good husband? Did I make us a good life? There were no confessions I heard—no call for the priest to seek forgiveness, no surprises for the epic ending of this novel.

Only recently has my reluctance to get transparency bothered me—I could have asked so much of her. All those years condensed into a few hours—she remained who she was until the end. I should not have been surprised. If I had a strong, really strong belief in my Catholic faith, I would wait for the answers when we see each other again in the next life. How I want to believe that—yet not delude myself. This belief implies a deity and Jesus. Philosopher Luc Ferry in *On Love* says it well: "If love is what gives meaning to our lives, what are we to do about death, which brings it [love] to a full stop?" And as we become less religious, with less faith, we are not sheltered by the conviction of resurrection, and the gloominess of death and the loss of love are more noticeable. And yet we love again…

There was a real change in Jane that evening after we said goodbye to Bill's family in Florida. This was the turning point where the dying process had taken its hold. She began to have belly pain and nausea and became weaker. She asked me to feel her abdomen. I had tried to make it a point to leave the doctoring to her doctors and had not examined her as a physician does. My God, I thought. Her liver was enlarged and tender—the likely cause of this pain. This cancer was relentless, and the tumor burden was becoming a crisis. She looked awful, but she didn't need to be seen at an ER or hospital. Let's get home, we thought early in the morning. And again, there was the question "How much? How much time do you think is left?" Maybe August, I thought. But I told her I thought she could make it through Christmas. Whether or not she believed me I don't know.

I did all the driving back to Charleston in one sitting. She slept all the way in the front seat without incident. She may require intravenous fluids, I thought, as her intake was becoming nil. The next few days, she went to the infusion center and got fluids. She seemed better. No crisis. She made a brief weekend trip to Chicago to see her father and Tom Croak, her longtime priest friend from Loyola, the place where she had received her MBA. I've seen pictures of her on that last visit—how the hell did she do it? She even talked about going back when she felt "better."

My daughter Joy came home the weekend before Jane died—she was even up for sewing something for my daughter, called her father to set up a visit for him with us, and even talked about us going to New York on July Fourth—a week away. There was no way in hell we were going to New York, and I thought her dad should come sooner than the time slot that had been set for three weeks ahead. Things were moving quickly. I did not say anything about her father's visit, but I told Jane I thought New York would be too much for her. She reluctantly agreed. Joy went back to school that Sunday. I had no reason to hold her back. It was to be Jane's last weekend.

Life can quickly falter and be taken from us. There was so little reserve for her to hold on to. I spoke with Susan Garfinkel that Monday to see if she would stay with Jane on Tuesday morning—the next day. She had a doctor's appointment, and I thought I could get home early afternoon to take her. I had not missed any work throughout her illness. I planned to take Wednesday, June 26, off. In a short time, her breathing was more labored and prohibited her movement from one room to another. When I got home that Tuesday to relieve Susan, it was obvious I would not be getting her up or down the stairs. We would cancel the doctor's visit—I saw little gain. Jane made it very clear she did not want to be hospitalized. I agreed. She had met with hospice and signed on the previous Friday.

As Good As It Gets

    I called hospice, and they sent a nurse that last Tuesday evening. This was the time to start morphine to try to slow her labored respirations and to taper the frightening feeling of air hunger. That midnight I went to an all-night CVS for liquid morphine. She was becoming more restless and anxious, but not confused. She needed rest and sleep. She had not eaten for the last two days. Rarely could she leave the bed, and she needed assistance to the bathroom. The hospice nurse left around 10:00 p.m.

    The morphine was bitter and not as easy as I'd thought to give her. At some point, though, she got some relief and smiled at me. Do you know how wonderful a small gesture like a smile can be? I still, if I think about it, can occasionally see that smile now. What a reward—a gift—that I was able to do something for her that was meaningful. There was no need for words here—language gets in the way. Just a touch, a hand held, an embrace as she tried to sleep. I felt helpless but didn't show it. I was afraid but didn't show the terror of feeling impotent. I listened through the night to the raspy sounds of her labored, heavy, noisy breathing, but she seemed to sleep. I don't remember needing to get up. I would be with her tomorrow. She could not be alone.

    Wednesday, June 26, 2013, was to be Jane's last day. It was really the only day of her entire illness that I took off from work to care for her. The shortness of breath was worse again. Jane was mildly anxious but alert and not confused. Papers had come for her to sign the New York apartment over to my name to avoid the obvious tax consequences if she died. She read every line, even with a yellow marker. I thought, Jane, this is not the time for this! Please, just sign the papers, and let's rest. I felt awful and guilty—how could this be? She could not find her breath and was now a little agitated. I suspect the lack of oxygen, dehydration, lack of eating, and added morphine all were contributing to this agitation, mild confusion, and worsening weakness. She wanted to find a "better," cooler room in the house where she could feel the air. All the fans were blowing at full speed. I had made a quick trip downstairs to take out my dogs, Max and Charlie. I heard a noise upstairs—she was struggling to go from one room to another. Holy shit! I ran upstairs to find her in the other bedroom, sitting on the floor, unable to get up. The breathing was definitely worse—more labored and faster. It took nearly twenty minutes to go from one bedroom to another bedroom.. I needed to give more morphine, but it was so bitter for her to swallow, and now even this was a challenge.

I was alone, and I felt really alone. I'm sure if I had called for help, Paul and Susan would have dropped everything and come. Susan was a chosen one Jane would let close to witness her frailty and dependency. I didn't call for help. I questioned my competency. Could I be doing a better job? I needed affirmation that I was doing the best I could do. In the short time of a single morning, she worsened. She hardly could stand anymore without me nearby. She moved constantly, looking for a comfortable place to breathe. I thought, Dear God, stay still! Rest. Close your eyes, Jane, if just for a few minutes.

I tried morphine again, but it was hard for her to take—so bitter. I tried some water—just water. How was I going to get through this day, and what about tonight? She refused any food—even broth would not go down. There were no hospice calls. I was not sure they could help with much more than what I was doing. I would have thought they would have at least checked up on me to see how I was managing. Dying at home is not what they make it sound like—this was hard. I would never see hospice in the same way for my patients. This required a village! More restlessness. Not enough morphine or too much morphine!

It was now noon. Maybe she seemed a bit quieter. I had added lorazepam (Ativan) along with her morphine, and maybe this combination had begun to work. Her dear and old friend, Judy, was on her way at Jane's request. Judy was an attorney whom Jane wanted to help with the kids' trust. Her flight from Baltimore would land around 4:00 p.m., and I was happy the prospect of extra eyes and hands. No calls from work. The kids were unaware of the changes, and I was trying to calculate in my head the timing of her last hours—were these her last hours, or days, or even longer, perhaps? Did I have enough medication? Should I try to feed her something? Should I call her oncologist, Rita? No calls. No hospice calls. Where were they? Was it because I was an oncologist, a death and dying physician, an expert? It was expected that I would know what to do and how to act. I was alone and needed to keep it together. My Jane was unrecognizable now—she was no longer that survivor but the summation of all that was good about life—no longer who she was, or wanted to be, or should be. I didn't hear God's name or voice—should I have called a priest to talk or pray for her? Was this my fault?

This is what real suffering looks like, I thought, although she would always deny that she suffered. Never did she ask to have something to make death come quicker, but only to help relieve her pain and air hunger. Jane and I would have discussions before she was ill about assisted suicide—she was always on the side of the person who chose to die if pain or life had become too much of a burden. She never asked for an easier death, though. I think she was able to find happiness while suffering.

She was up and on the move again—now close to 1:00 p.m. Time had slowed—every movement in slow motion. The room was quite bright. It was a warm and sunny June day. The temperature was comfortable. The dogs were downstairs, quiet and resting. She suddenly jerked up out of the bed. Her mantra all morning had been "It's not your fault! It's not your fault!" This was another gift for me to hold on to—even now the refrain offers comfort. Last words, I think. I believe she knew I tried my best. It was difficult being the breast oncologist, watching from a distance and living with it so near me. I was the full professor, the palliative care specialist, and so unable to make things better. I had run out of words—there was no language to pass comfort on to her. It was what it was, and it was dreadful!

She arose and moved up very fast—it surprised me she had that amount of energy. "I have to go to the bathroom. I have to go!" I held her up, and suddenly she cried out, "I can't catch my breath! I can't breathe." She went limp and collapsed in my arms; her eyes rolled up, and she fell unconscious. No further words. I carried her the short distance to our bed. It was over. I had lost her, here and now and forever. Shallow breathing and then nothing. Jane was no more. I wanted someone else in that room, at that time, to be with me—but alone I was. No one should die alone. Sister Amata had realized that long ago—we should not be abandoned. The lone witness to death should also not be alone. Judy would arrive too late. I walked downstairs. The thermostat had a yellow sticky note from Jane: "Keep the temperature at 68 degrees." I observed.

Jane and I had been married on June 29, 1993. I was alone with her the afternoon she died almost twenty years to the day later—June 26, 2013. It was not a surprise, just sooner than I had expected.

Watching someone die over a protracted time creates shadows on the present. You live in a foggy past and a grieved future all at the same time. You try to picture events in the future without the lost individual you loved—you know the end is coming, yet at the same time you can vividly recall bits and tidbits of something that keeps the dead person alive and relevant for the present. It's all a terrible game the mind plays.

There is also something about the aesthetics of dying that makes us humans leave this earthly existence not looking very good. Maybe that's why "young men fear death and old men fear dying." We become fearful of what we've seen or heard from others—the unwanted hideous potential nature of ourselves when it all comes crashing in. Our bodies become unfamiliar to us, and we notice ourselves as outcasts in our mirrors. The dying shy away from others, for they have entered the separated world of the truly ill—no more visitors here. The dying process starts an accelerated fast track to aging—muscle mass fades, cheekbones disappear, no buttocks remain to show off, and there is a stench of frailty that prevails. We are no longer the person we knew, and we wonder if our place in life among the well is altered so much that we have lost all worth. It is difficult to appear this way as an ill person and hard as hell for a loved one to witness the unwanted modifications of a body they no longer recognize. It reminds us, including the physician, all too well that this could be us. And even if not now, it could happen tomorrow. I remember that when I was a young physician in the days when hospital reimbursement allowed patients to stay unchallenged in their hospital beds, they would bring to their hospital rooms reminders of home and themselves: flowers, greeting cards, and personal photographs of themselves—younger, prettier, more fit and healthy. The message, to me, the doctor, was clear—this person today in this bed is not the only me. That person in that photo has a history and a past story that was real and good—and had value and worth.

I submit that it may be harder to endure when the deterioration happens in patients in their prime and with promising futures. But no matter what age we are, we wish to be seen changing at a pace that is graceful, where we have some faint gift of ownership—perhaps a shared alteration of ourselves with others—a collective remembrance of what we all looked like. Montaigne would echo this: "Whoever saw old age, that did not applaud the past, and condemn the present times?" Samuel Beckett once said that the day we die is another ordinary day, just shorter.

I also wonder if the changes seen and made by the ravages of illness can make it easier to let that life go—and one can pray for death to come and be the friend of the dying. My mom was always concerned about her appearance to others—neat, clean, put together, and proper. She perished over time via the majestic savage wasting of advanced pancreatic cancer. If you don't or cannot eat, and you vomit over weeks repeatedly, you will not look the same, and you will certainly not look well. By the time her death came at 2:00 a.m. on Thanksgiving in 1999, she was unrecognizable to me as my mom. She was a frail, pathetic corpse of her former self, and it was obviously time for me to let her go. Please, God, take her, I prayed, and relieve her and me of this pain and suffering. I should note that I rarely recall this awful scene, and yet I remember a mosaic portrait of her: my mom as a young woman when I was a young boy, and simultaneously a picture of a mature woman when my children were young—all blended, melted into one picture.

Lucy Grealy, an award-winning poet, wrote beautifully about the aesthetics of illness and treatment in a memoir called *Autobiography of a Face*. She speaks eloquently about the pain of disfigurement caused by our relentless battle to rid patients of their diseases. We physicians can mutilate body and soul with the best of them—mastectomies, amputations, ingenious bodily diversions—as well as add to depression, impotency, and sterility. She states clearly, "I spent five years of my life being treated for cancer, but since then I've spent fifteen years being treated for nothing other than looking different from everyone else. It was the pain from that, from feeling ugly, that I always viewed as the great tragedy of my life. The fact that I had cancer seemed minor in comparison."

I believe the awful aesthetics of dying create an environment that worsens the natural separation of the dying person from all others who are seen as well. This, I must confess, also includes the physician and the caretakers of the sick person. And through it all, the person as patient is calling out to us, reminding us they are not dead but are still alive and living among us. It may seem counterintuitive, but only when the imminence of death's finality is finally acknowledged and recognized, if not accepted, can there be some peace and openness—perhaps closure. This is what Hans Zinsser describes as a "cancer understanding."

Illness truly rips apart the normal harmony of the interconnecting of our human lives. All of us must try not to turn our backs on the aesthetics of the dying but instead try to embrace the rich opportunity to share a life in the most profound of times. But, I submit, it is not an easy task. We must see through a different lens. Jane was dead.

As Good As It Gets

I was not all right. There was this awkward sense of relief that it was over. The war against cancer had been fought and lost, but it had been fought hard and with dignity. She had died as she wanted, in her own bed. We had talked weeks before, and she had told me quite clearly that she was content with the life that she lived. There was no incompleteness for her. She'd do it all the same way. One can suffer and be happy.

Jane had made it easy for me—always told me clearly what she needed and wanted. Her inner thoughts were hers alone: Where am I going? How does this all end? More importantly, she made it very clear there should be no viewing of her dead body—no prolonged wake, but a memorial service with those she knew and cared about. She wanted to be cremated quickly, and her ashes could go wherever I thought best. She died on a Wednesday—the cremation was set for Friday. The house was now filled with friends, the kids, and Judy, who arrived two hours after Jane died. I had given a dress to the funeral home in case the kids wanted to see her again. We gathered together Friday morning, and no one wanted to remember her as a corpse. I made certain they were sure, as there could be no going back on this decision. "No" was the response. Her dad called and wanted me to take a photo of Jane before cremation. But why? I recalled a photograph of Jane's family together at her mother's casket from years before. I couldn't do this to Jane. I still have my text to her father:

June 29, 2013, 2:37 p.m.
Dick,

This was a difficult morning for all of us. When it came time for us to go, we couldn't. Jane so wanted her dignity and we wanted both to honor her wishes and remember her to each in our own way. I made sure that they were comfortable with their decision and had closure. My thoughts are constantly with her.
—Frank

It was over.

I've come to realize that we do treat the dead better than the living. At least publicly, we seem to show more reverence to a dead body or cremated ashes. This is especially evident if the deceased died sacrificing their life for something greater than themselves. For the fallen soldier, even unknown, we display enormous devotion and composure. The dead remain silent about these gestures of heroism we give them for just dying. Are they in a better place? Are they anyplace? Are they able to witness our offerings, or is it just show? It doesn't seem to matter, does it? I will continue to act to the dead as if it matters, because it does. The hearse always will go first, and the cars will follow.

There is no grave site to visit or place to bring flowers to or for her remains. I have the essence of her with me in the next room, under my work table. She had given me no preferences about where to place her ashes: "It doesn't matter—I leave it to you." I kept them close to me for nearly a year—did they belong along the South Carolina coast, in the Northwest, where she sailed in her twenties, by the beach of the Isle of Palms she loved so much? Did I do this with the kids—make it a family outing? In the end, I gave the ashes to her father to place near her mom back in her beloved Indiana—where her father joined her finally. He was content and happy to have something of his daughter again. I was numb, unmoved—sad that she was no longer with me—but it was, in the end, some relief and closure that I did a decent thing.

Jane was cremated on June 28, 2013. I had purchased an urn and kept her ashes—really a misnomer because what remains is broken-down bone fragments and maybe some minerals and salts. No matter, this was the stuff of her life, which I had known well and loved, and for me, they evoked personal meaning and memories. It was a vestibule to those memories anytime I wanted or needed them. In those early days after her death, her ashes remained close to me under my desk. It was difficult to run free of past times with her when she was so damn near at all times.

Jane grew up in Hamden, Indiana. Her father and two brothers were still living there, along with old friends and family who knew her well. We planned to return to celebrate her

Catholic funeral mass that July. No wants or *don'ts* were passed down, and I was struck by her indifference to what would happen to her leftover remains. I would know what was best to do. There were no requests to fly and drop her ashes in the ocean. Hawaii, a place she loved, did not make the list. I didn't have to climb any hills, or God forbid, reach a mountain peak to scatter her about.

    I had no idea regarding the protocol for cremated ashes at the airport. I didn't want a frenzy of issues the day we were to travel to Chicago. My youngest daughter and I decided to go to the Charleston International Airport and inquire about the rules for ashes. I spoke with the TSA agents, and they understood my nervousness and awkwardness about what should happen. The message was simple—don't worry; leave it to them for tomorrow. They would be there and get Jane's remains to the gate for our United Airlines flight to Chicago.

    Our flight was set for 10:00 a.m. on July 11, 2013, with United. Joy and Matthew would accompany me, and we would meet up with everyone in Chicago. The mass was set for 10:30 a.m. on Saturday, July 13. I carried the box with the urn to the TSA checkpoint. The attendant remembered me and noted that they would get her through for us. To my surprise, the conveyer belt let off the luggage and then stopped. No new pieces would be allowed on the conveyer. People were asked to stay in place. With quiet awe, I placed the box on the empty belt, and alone she moved through for the screen. It was done with grace and reverence for someone who was a stranger. A stranger who had celebrity status only to me. I must confess I cried. I wept for an act of kindness to someone I knew and loved deeply. I thanked them all, and we boarded. Because the box was too large to fit under the seat, Jane not only got to fly first class, but she also flew with the pilots in the cockpit. We were escorted off the plane first, and again people waited for us. She would have liked that.

    I was quite relieved it all went so well. Frank, you pulled it off, I thought. It was good that my younger children witnessed such kindness and human connectedness. There should be respect for the dead—it is a human endeavor we practice because a life matters. It's important to have not only a good death but also a good send-off. The hearse always goes first—the cars follow.

This wonderful human experience of love's bond, no doubt, rewarded me with a profound sense of gaining meaning for my life. My life was enriched and tightly woven, connected to the wants and needs of another. I had suffered when she had pain and rejoiced when there was laughter to share. And this was different from the bonds with my grandmother, my parents, and even my children. Nozick states it well: "The people you love are included inside your boundaries, their well-being is your own." There is an ontological transformation that love gives birth to—the immense interconnecting of lives and all that implies, an identity of oneness. We file more than a joint tax return—we file as an ontological human partnership that itself has character, separate from each as an individual. It is an intimate and close bond wrapped up in mutual affirmation and trust of each other. That's what makes it so hard when the bond is severed—especially by the permanence of death. It is no more and cannot be anymore. More, it had its own life—developed, reorganized, readjusted to the change of what life offers, for "better or worse." Most of us, I suspect, feel, at the time we say these words, that it can't get much better than this, and we have no clue about how much worse it can be. Can the "we" undertake the worst of our tomorrows no matter what life tosses at us? In the end, one can acknowledge a happy life.

In the end, one can admit to a life of happiness and meaning and value and completeness—realizing that, looking it over in reverse, one would not alter the outcome of this human bond. I am finally left unwanting. God only knows I would have wanted more of life with Jane, but it was as good as it could get. And in the end, I'm grateful. The Harvard Study of Adult Development, which was initiated in 1938, tells it clearly—the good life and happiness are tied not to our genes, money, social class, or intelligence but to having loved ones to rely upon and talk with. I must confess, I was not cheated!

Julian Barnes rewarded me with words of insight after Jane died. The year Jane passed, in 2013, Barnes released *Levels of Life*, about the death of his wife, Pat Kavanagh, whom he married in 1978. I had recently lost Jane, and the pain of loss was fresh. He wrote about what I was missing, "the longing for something or someone." I was missing the very essence of someone whom I spoke with every day, shared each meal with, and closed my eyes for sleep nightly next to her body. And yet, as expected, time unfailingly moves to another day and season, and you remain. The wonderful solitude of life does begin to mitigate the longing, and the necessary practice of living begins to heal. I'm never cured of this loss, but better.

This was not supposed to be our ending—we had never planned for or imagined this total separation from each other. And yet here was the reality of the situation: I was alone, Jane was gone, and all I had—given to me—was an urn with her ashes inside. It was difficult to fathom such a life bound in laughter, talent, and smarts compacted down to this urn, which I could put under my desk. I thought, Is this all there is? Is this as good as it gets?

Ah, but it is only now that I can answer the question posed: "Is this all there is?" The ashes are a by-product of life—the part that evolves, changes, ages, dies, and decays. We treat them with incredible diligence and respect even when they're under a desk, but what remain, quite alive, are vivid, ongoing, persistent memories and recollections of words, laughter, moments of delicate reflection, music, and harmonies of better times—my name spoken. And we live on and on until we are no longer visited in remembrances and thoughts—when our names and voices are no longer uttered and we become part of the cosmic mystery. And all suffering and pain are gone. George Gadow, a philosopher, rightly declares, "The frequent question, 'What is the meaning of my life?' can be interpreted…as a search for who will now share meaning with me." This persistent, constant loss of deep connection to one another—this suffering—is part of our human drama and reality, but, again as Gadow notes, "pure rationality is as meaningless as pure pain." I don't want to lose my human connection and interpersonal meaning. My Jane lives in me. I don't need the ashes any longer.

It really is hard watching a loved one suffer the ravages and indignity of overwhelming illness. How she wondered how this all would come to an end—most of us don't dwell on that last breath, but the timebound do. Jane would often, very often, recall watching her grandfather die a respiratory death and admit how afraid she was of that kind of ending. And yet, indeed, that's what we got. The cosmic universe doesn't give a shit about what we think or want. I must confess I don't think any prayer would have made it easier or taken it away. My God—we pray to a deity that didn't rid the world of suffering for us but joined in the suffering.

We often had conversations about assisted suicide—Jane pro and me against it. But she *never* asked me to help her die—only relieve her pain and make her breathing easier. That's how the morphine came to be there that last night. Don't believe those doubts were with me—I gave her enough to rid her of the dyspnea and tachypnea (two great Greek words) but not cause her death. God forbid—I had enough angst and guilt; I didn't need that added. Plus, I was alone. It's not good to be alone!

Jane lost her cancer battle around 1:30 p.m. that early summer, Wednesday afternoon, June 26, 2013. She was an avid reader, a great partner to edit whatever I wrote. She would make changes with her red marker, making corrections and always improving whatever I thought was satisfactory and ready to be submitted. She was a stickler for good grammar and punctuation, and eventually, I got used to her insightful editorial criticism. Months after she passed away, I was separating her stuff and my stuff to stay or be discarded when I discovered in the corner of the bookcase a small blue worn-down notebook that had the word "thoughts" handwritten on the inner cover. I had not seen this book before, nor did she ever admit to me that she was writing or keeping any record of her experience with chemotherapy or facing the awful truth that she was going to die. I have read this small book more times than I can ever count—alone. It keeps her alive. I have never shared it with anyone. She never gave me instructions to read it aloud or to impart its simple wisdom from somebody dying who was so freaking smart and insightful about her ultimate fate. It was obviously started when the disease was realized to be an unrelenting, progressive stage IV—and she knew it would kill her.

So when I read what she wrote, I take it seriously because it comes from someone who paved the way for all who must follow. She did it with grace and courage. We should consider and absorb simple wisdom and authenticity. Some of her notations include the following:

February 4, 2012 [two months after the biopsy-proven cancer recurred]

"It's different this time…" That's what I say when people ask me how I'm doing with the Big C.

May 5, 2012

I feel love…for all the wonderful people who have sworn their support and their loyalty and shared their encouragement and humor and comfort.

Love for my children—no bitterness, no hurt, no regrets…just love!

Love for Frank, who tries each day to let me know he's on my side and will do whatever he can to ease my pain as this new stage of chemo begins, knowing it will not be easy but hoping for the best, despite the odds.

Love for Dad, who knows me best and my family.

July 12, 2012

Courage doesn't always roar. Sometimes courage is the little voice at the end of the day, that says "I'll try again tomorrow."

Hope whispers: "One more time."

And now, chemo again!

Summer 2012

Hair…
What use?
What vanity…

*I like hats, always have.
And yet,
this time around,
I can't bear to lose it...strand by strand
until just a soft halo is left.
Still, I won't let it go!
Not this time.
Why was it fun and so entertaining the first time around—a night of crazy hairdo, then the final shave and goodbye. Voilà !
Change of perspective...
(It's fun being an alien to neighbor kids!)*

September 2012

Perhaps that is hope? What an abstract word, concept. Different times, varied events and circumstances lead to hope...from the most basic child's hope for a bike on Christmas, all the way to "hope against hope"—which is the crux of the matter for many cancer patients suffering with terminal cancer. Lexicographers describe it as "having hope," though it seems to be baseless.

But all definitions of the word have a common thing: expectation of <u>some</u> good that is yet to be.

November 2012

*Worry...negative prayer
"We are spiritual beings having a human experience."—Pierre Teilhard de Chardin
(Doesn't that sound so perfectly correct?)*

January–February 2013

"Only a few know my secret. I don't think I can bear the eyes of the many; and so, they are few. At least for now..."

February 2013, NYC

"Time spent laughing is time spent with the gods. Laughing and crying—it's the same relief."—Joni Mitchell

Humor is the instrument for taking pain playfully.

As Good As It Gets

Writer: Woody Allen / Teacher + liver: Frank Brescia

Sometimes, but only some, I feel as if my life is the eye of a hurricane.

Easy...no!

Possible...perhaps.

I enjoy the little things...There are so many of them.

The only thing I need to finish by tomorrow is today.

December 2012

Write a letter in the dark of night...read it in daylight, then send it, or destroy it. Try to let go of why it was written at all. Is this forgiveness?

January 2013

And suddenly, without the smallest warning, the probability of not existing takes shape. I feel it. How odd it comes so quietly while preparing another's life to begin...to have the challenge of letting go on so many levels, simultaneously. Is there a master plan?

June 11, 2013 [15 days before her death]

The simple act of taking a breath...how much we take it for granted, we humans...until it's not so simple, nor easy...

Is this how it might end? It will be a struggle to triumph against the frazzled edges of a guild made over a lifetime of joy, love, loss, success, heartbreaks, awakening, challenges, searching for the best I've given, the pain endured, the questions unanswered, the magic of understanding purpose...What differences have I made from my tapestry?

The calm can turn to chaos,
Serene can become stormy,
Giggles can turn to moans,
Futures can seem limited.
As a new reality sneaks into my psyche (go away!!),
Stealing away my dreams

Of years to come and adventures in the dreams… not yet realized.

Yet doubt finds its way in…what about the kids? And siblings? They have their own lives…let them live, some worry about me…and yet, I recall my own anger at Vera (mother) and Dad when we realized they had hidden the seriousness of her illness. Could we have done anything to ease their burden?

I always wondered…could they do anything to ease mine, if they knew? Perhaps just a tiny bit of empathy…is that worth the price of their peace of mind and security of my being here? Will they also be angry?

March 2013

Real fear is something quite new to me…the questions…it starts with anxiety—mainly for others, but occasionally for me, as well…Fear that I haven't said enough of the right things; I haven't shown the best of me; I haven't given enough of my time, my mind, myself to the people and causes I truly believe in. Have I been the very best cheerleader possible? Have I planted the best and most lasting seeds in my garden of life…will they continue to bloom where I've planted them in children, family, friends, and loved ones?

Favor: give me the gesture and gift…please take those seeds and plant them in your own life gardens and see what happens! Good things mostly.

Courage doesn't always roar. Sometimes courage is the little voice at the end of the day that says "I'll try again tomorrow."

March 2013

But I can't worry about my days being numbered when I know I've already lived forever: over a lingering dinner at Highlands Sur, Carmel; breathless, as I ski down a slope with my children and friends; walking the streets of large and tiny towns, no matter the languages spoken, always smiling and often surprised at how easily people communicate; riding camels and dune buggies with Joy and Matt in Egypt; Frank—strolling the streets of Berlin, Amsterdam, Paris, Rome, Taormina, San Fran, New York, and so many fantastic cities, each with its own flavor, eating our way to new heights...

One-on-one holidays with so many friends and family over the years...

So many giggles, oohs and aahs, and awe: always the <u>awe</u> in travel...waterfalls, flowers as large as Frisbees, fireworks that light up the sky and the heart, but not the best for me, not people I love.

If I'm going to wait for the gasping for breath to take me, why not just give in? Saying yes to giving in would be easy, but who loves <u>that</u>? Not me. If I'm going to fight for what and those I love, I must get up and get going...until I just cannot...Who knows when that will be? It's not a bucket list—it's a challenge I'll take for as long as I'm able and include as many people and places as I can—even farewells can be filled with awe; I'll make some new memories and revisit some old...laughter, silliness, sadness, and joyous times...mostly. And I'll see how time allows me this plan of mine!

The greatest dignity to be found in death is the dignity of the life that preceded it. This is a form of hope we can all achieve. Hope lives in the meaning of what our lives have been and being reminded of that at the end of life.

A promise a caregiver can give and keep is the certainty that no man nor woman will be left alone to die. It is the promise of spiritual companionship near the end that gives us final hope when none exists; a tranquil comfort, easing of a patient's departure, by hastening the moments of death...the "good death" by any definition.

August 6, 2012

Suffering is <u>not</u> the same as unhappiness. I'm learning that the moment for myself can be put off indefinitely...until the possibility dissolves, as it will...if I blink.

Frank J. Brescia

Am I willing to grab these precious moments? The decision is mine alone.

I believe...

Even if I've only helped change the world in the life of one person, I have, in my small way, changed the world. I'm so happy to have done that with my life. I have made a difference.

Even though this life has been difficult, I consider it an honor to have lived it; to have loved the people I have known; to have learned so much about so many; to have been loved, despite my imperfections and frailties.

PART VI:
Postdeath Reflections

Dr. Thomas Smith, an oncologist at Johns Hopkins, wrote about what the dean at Yale Medical School thought the incoming medical students should possess as prerequisites for admission. These requirements included the following: (1) having lived in a foreign country without knowing the language; (2) having loved, truly loved, someone deeply; and (3) having faced, at some point in life, their mortality.

It was time for me to face the fact of loss and mourn. It was time to grieve. With grief, there is often the companion guilt. They commonly run together as a couple, knocking at the door. What could I have done better? Had I done enough? Should I have sought other opinions? Had I comforted her enough? Were my words helpful? I needed to let Jane's elderly father know he had lost his daughter—he too had suffered the loss of his wife to breast cancer at the same age of sixty-two. My kids, away at school, would need to come home. How difficult to tell them their mother was dead on the phone without holding them and seeing their faces. They knew treatments had stopped but, like me, had failed to realize the closeness of time. Perhaps I could have been a better communicator regarding time—always a better historian than a prophet. Her death to me was like the last sentence of an epic novel. I had read that analogy once from literary critic James Wood of the *New Yorker*. In a book, however, we can reopen the pages and start the life again. I would need to relive images in memories that were so fragile and often wrong. We tend to cut away all the bad stuff and struggles. People close to us really alter our lives in many ways, and we are changed—me, for the better. I, indeed, had changed with Jane, and now I felt, for a time, very alone.

The death of a loved one changes the landscape of possibilities—causes a pause, a rebooting of life, of what comes next. And there is this terrible thing called grief. But one has to eat, go to work, pay the bills, prepare the taxes, talk with the children, and have some meaningful and not-so-meaningful conversations. Forge ahead through the immediacy of what needs doing, like going through probate, figuring out what to keep and what to discard. I had the luxury of time and no real commitments. The kids were settled or in school. I owned little—my car, my furniture, my clothes, so I had the freedom to consider my next steps. My children wanted me to move back to New York—but it was too cold, too damn expensive, and most of all, too close to them! The hard part was trying to sleep alone in the marital bed of a lifetime. I missed the sounds of in-and-out breathing—the sound of life. I missed her smell and movement.

Jane's death removed the close bond of our lives, which had been so interwoven that there was no longer a "we" (i.e., Jane and Frank) but an "I" alone. Except for the multiple hidden messages from the grave, I didn't have to seek affirmation or permission from her or anyone for anything. There was no "What do you want for dinner? What movie do you want to watch tonight?" Everything seemed open, and time just slowed down. All was gray, no Technicolor here. Quiet and slower. No mumbling of sounds or voices in another room. I kept the temperature at sixty-eight degrees. I had what is described by

Julian Barnes as the "rust of the soul." I would stay put, here in this rented house, for now, but not forever. I was seventy-one years old and a widower. My heart was broken.

The "how" of what happened was easy to explain. She was a woman, over fifty, with a mother with a history of breast cancer. The more fundamental question was why. Cancer because of being a woman, genetics, too much estrogen, not enough estrogen, having lived near nuclear waste? I don't ever recall Jane asking why. That's Job's question, isn't it? She voiced much more acceptance or resignation than I have felt. She was outspoken about telling me she had lived the life she wanted to live—had few meaningful regrets, had deep, long, loving friendships, and had found happiness. Her nervousness seemed more about leaving such an incompetent person as I behind. She had doubts I could be trusted to go on without her. I was an idiot! I knew the "How does this happen?" question too well. The "Why?" question still hung out there for me.

I had seen so much of death in a lifetime, starting from my childhood Bronx tribal home—grandparents, parents, close friends, soldiers, and beloved dogs. This was different. They told me her loss would be different. This time it was near to breaking my soul—no boundaries here. I really hurt. My close friends saw my pain and bewilderment. I had a newly acquired social awkwardness. I'd rather stay at home alone. I had reached an age where all those who knew me back to my childhood—who really knew me as little Frankie—were no longer here. There was no one to question or seek comfort from. That train had left the station long ago. I thought, You're on your own, and you better get used to this. You're the senior citizen here and now. Don't look for comfort from your elders, because they are not here anymore, and even if they were, looking for answers from that group, which couldn't answer basic things way back then, is even more ridiculous. You're grieving because you lost something of great value to you—something meaningful—and it's permanently lost and forever gone. It's no more. Only an urn filled with ashes remains. Is this the product of a life? The more it's worth, the heavier the hurt. And you're asking why?

There was never a request to get second and third opinions. Jane either accepted her situation or trusted me to navigate her course of treatment and options. I tried to talk to my friends around the country whom I trusted and from whom I sought out affirmation that what was being done was what they would recommend. I trusted Lisa Carey's assessment of Jane's disease and available options. She just had a bad disease. There were no attempts or requests to go to Fatima or seek faith healers or unorthodox therapies. She had done her homework. Her disease was relentless, with no hint of a response to anything thrown at it. What had been brewing those nearly eight years? Jane kept her spiritual beliefs close to herself—she had been brought up, like me, as a Roman Catholic, though without the Italian flavor of voodooism thrown in. She wouldn't engage with me when I asked about what she thought about God, an afterlife, miracles, or seeking spiritual curative therapies. She would look at me when I tried to ask, and she would just smile at me. The truth was, I had seen miracles in my practice that I couldn't explain. No miracles, however, were here for me or for my Jane.

My empathy for the spouses of my patients became much closer because of my experience with Jane. It was the struggle to say the right thing to enhance comfort and not be an asshole. The question "How are you feeling?" was no longer a meaningful question. "What can I do?" was better. I advised myself: Make sure your demeanor is right—not too serious or grim. Can you instill encouragement? Hope died a long time before this final curtain. When to smile? When is there an appropriate joke? Should I bring up the banal duties of daily living? Should I stay home, work, come home early, get help, call friends for help, let the children be aware of the downward progression? I could feel death's presence in the room. I grieved and wondered over and over: Could I have done better? Could I have changed the course of this battle? For God's sake, I'm a breast oncologist, a palliative care "expert," a reasonably good physician—and I was so lost in doubt and guilt. Guilt and grief blended together. I felt for my patients' spouses, sisters, mothers and fathers, children—for I had visited their world.

I had imagined often that Jane could get better—that somehow the cancer would respond to something. In the past, in my practice, I had seen people's diseases just appear to get tired and stop growing, and life would go on. I wished I had deeper faith in God and that I could witness some miracle, but I prayed less, became more doubtful of a merciful divine spirit, and held to the truth of what was to be. I don't know if Jane prayed or if she wanted me to pray more for her. The subject never came up between us. Should we have spoken more about God and faith or what was next for us?

In my practice, it was not uncommon for the patient to fail the prescribed treatment—often physicians even used the awful terminology of Jane's having "failed to respond to the chemotherapy." I've seen families place insidious blame on their loved ones for not considering the power of positive thinking. One quickly realizes how much of medicine—at least the kind of medicine I deal with—is such a spiritual endeavor, a spiritual act of practice. I wanted the God I doubted, the God I no longer prayed to, somehow now to intervene. I so want to believe that there is a sustenance of hope that there is an after consciousness where we can once again "meet" and have the experience of mutual presence. Can that really be? I'm asking for the absurdity of certainty of the possibility of this being part of our ultimate reality—a consciousness beyond the grave. I'm asking for the absurdity that life, in the end, has some meaning and reverence given by the cosmos and perhaps by a divine being.

There is no question that death makes the act of living matter more. If immortal, I have time to change my mind and time to admit to my failures, and I have ample time to wait. With death at my front doorway, I don't have any time to lose, and I have little time for regret. I may be cheated in life's future adventures or cheated about past mistakes, but there is only a limited time frame in which to seek forgiveness or peace.

Maybe Hamlet's question is off and it's not "To be or not to be," but rather "How to be or not be." Our timebound lives also limit the horror of ongoing pain and existential anxiety that haunts so many of our lives. We ultimately need and seek refuge in peace. And then we rest. It is an eternal rest. Will God awaken us?

A brief story: Daniel was a patient I met in the summer of 1999. He was forty-five years old, married with two small children, and otherwise healthy. He presented that late spring with worsening abdominal pain, weight loss, tiredness, and then jaundice—a turn of the body to yellow. A workup unfortunately quickly discovered that he had a pancreatic mass and a diagnosis of pancreatic cancer. This is a devastating illness with a five-year survival rate of less than 5 percent for all comers. A small percentage of newly diagnosed even are offered surgery because the cancer becomes either locally advanced or metastatic to the liver. Often, because of anatomical positioning, it blocks the biliary duct, and jaundice occurs.

Daniel was considered operable, and that August he was offered a Whipple procedure by Dr. Paul Baron, an oncology surgeon. Not surprisingly, when opened, he was found to have extensive intra-abdominal disease. A biliary bypass was performed to relieve the obstruction, and he was closed. A course of chemotherapy (gemcitabine) plus radiation was offered, but he quickly progressed, with new disease seen on CT scans of the abdomen. He could not work, had constant pain requiring oxycodone regularly around the clock, and was losing weight because he couldn't eat well. He had constant nausea. He was on his way to die, and he was aware of the gravity of the situation.

We had a clinical trial to offer—three drugs: cisplatin, gemcitabine (which he had already tried), and IV irinotecan—none of these drugs alone is easy to take. This was also an early drug trial with little real hope that this would make a difference in the picture presented to us. By late January 2000, he had completed a few doses, had severe neutropenia (dangerously low white blood cells), and required admission to our hospital because of a severe infection he had developed in his hand after accidentally hitting it with a hammer. Antibiotics were given, the hand required surgery, and he was discharged, better, to resume our chemotherapy at a lower dosage. Further chemotherapy became more difficult because of his blood counts, but he was feeling a little better—going to work one or two days per week, taking less oxycodone, and gaining weight. Staging scans in early spring were stable.

In May, Daniel was moderately improved—off oxycodone, and back to work,. He planned a trip with his wife in June, 2000 to visit Medjugorje where the Virgin Mary appeared and performed healing miracles first seen to children in 1981. I thought it seemed reasonable for him to go. In late May, the staging scans showed no visible cancer. We were elated, especially since his blood counts made it very difficult to keep a timely schedule of chemotherapy. I suggested that we have more extensive testing done when he returned from Europe. He was off treatment and feeling well when he returned home and to my office that summer. He told me he felt a "presence" of healing by the Blessed Mary before we completed a battery of tests which showed no malignancy in his body. I called Dr. Baron and asked, "Paul, remember Mr. D.?" I gave him the details to his delight. Repeat surgery? Was he really free of cancer, or if there was cancer still present, could it now be removed?

Daniel's wife had concerns about offending the deity and Mary, or both. She worried that they didn't have enough faith to leave things alone. I pushed to do the surgery to indeed show the miracle that had been accomplished. Surgery proved there was no cancer, and for over ten years, with repeated scans being done each year, he lived and was pancreatic cancer–free. Daniel was able to work with no issues.

One morning many years later, his wife called me. I had not seen Dan for several years. She said to me, "Dan seems to be missing steps and has fallen a few times." Nothing more. No abdominal pain. No weight loss. No jaundice. I suggested we see him in the clinic and examine him, especially since I had not seen him in a long time. When I examined him, I noted weakness of his muscle strength on one side of his body. He had also noted mild headaches that had started recently. An MRI of the brain showed what appeared to be a brain tumor—probably totally separate from his previous pancreatic cancer. Surgery confirmed a malignancy. Despite undergoing surgery, radiation, and chemotherapy, Dan was dead within a year and a half. He was grateful for the extra years, did not seem bitter, and was not angry at the Virgin Mary. I thought about Macbeth's words: "Life's but a walking shadow, a poor player that struts and fret his hour upon the stage and then is heard no more. It is a tale told by an idiot, full of sound and fury, signifying nothing."

Is this a message to Daniel or me or to both of us? It reminds me of the Middle Eastern folktale called "Appointment in Samarra," where a wealthy man and his servant are in the marketplace in Baghdad. The servant comes to his master and says, "I've seen Death in the market. Our eyes met, and I'm frightened. Please, I beg of you to give me one of your fastest horses, and I will go to the next town, Samarra." Death is in the person of a woman dressed in black. The master commits the horse to his servant, and he goes off. The wealthy man is now curious, and he himself confronts Death with a question: "Why have you frightened my servant so much?" Death replies, "I don't know why he was so frightened because I don't have an appointment with him until tomorrow in Samarra."

Dan's case did give me pause. What had happened here with this obviously religious man, who believed, along with his wife, that a miracle had happened? He had had all the symptoms, signs, pathology, and surgical staging observations that indicated he had a fatally progressive disease. There was no doubt. We had given this chemotherapy combination to others with the same disease—yet they died. The surgeon had opened and closed him, almost a year to the day—he was disease-free. He would have to die of something else at a later time—if he had dreams to work on, the time was on loan, borrowed time, so to speak. One could state that he seemed to be getting better prior to his trip to Europe, but he still possessed enormous faith that he could be healed by spiritual blessing. I have no way to confirm or deny that conviction—it is wonderful to see real faith do something positive.

For a scientist or a doubter, no way was this a miracle—a "God of the gaps" scenario. One could postulate that when he had the infection and sepsis, there was an overwhelming bodily immune response, akin to what is seen in the work and theory of Dr. William B Coley, who had reported numerous cases of tumor regression after massive infections. Possible? I don't know. Had I seen that before? Yes, once in a man I treated who had chronic lymphatic leukemia and was on chemotherapy and steroids—both immunosuppressive drugs. He was in the US Army Reserve as a cook at Fort Dix in New Jersey. He didn't want the army to know his medical status. He showed up for summer duty and got, like everyone else at the time, a smallpox vaccine—a live virus. He quickly developed disseminated vaccinia, sepsis with *Pseudomonas*. It was only after a serious infection that the progressive multiple skin pox lesions stopped progressing—there were no new lesions, and he began to heal.

Perhaps it was faith plus the infection plus my drugs. I never spoke to any clergy member or religious person about Dan—I'm not sure what such a person would conclude. Nobody needed to be made a saint after this miracle—that's often required for a new saint. The Blessed Mary didn't need the publicity. I honestly don`t know why he was healed.

Was this a conflict between science and religion? Pope John Paul II said it best: "Religion is not to tell us how heaven is made, but only how to get there." Did I become more religious? Should I have been more respectful of a miracle? How should I have incorporated this case into my practice? Why didn't he live a longer life—die when he was really old? There is the "Why?" question again. This second disease set the reality that I had or should have known—I don't prevent death but just substitute a new, different cause at a later time. I just wanted to have more time with Jane- just more precious time.

My grandmother Rose had explained to me a long time ago that the reason we had death was very simple. It was because of original sin. It was in Genesis from the Bible. Adam and Eve had everything they needed—it was paradise. There was no rain, hunger, pain, fear of death—the animals even talked. Adam and Eve lacked for nothing. I remember asking her, "Not even having to go to the bathroom?" It seemed such a waste (no pun) of time and energy to me. "No," she replied. I was angry, but more confused by this story. - Why? How? What could have motivated these idiots to not listen to God and eat the stupid fruit instead—even more, to listen to a snake? It may have been a fig or a grape—not even an apple. Maybe they should have eaten the snake! And what was this business concerning good and evil? We have death because of original sin. That's when we first faced our mortality.

The best description of and explanation for the fall of man that I ever read comes from the undertaker, writer, and poet Thomas Lynch. In his book *Bodies in Motion and at Rest*, there is a chapter called "Bible Studies." It's all there—why didn't I get it before? He notes, "They're not going to die, so why bother breeding? There's an endless supply and thus little demand…what's missing is heartache and desire, lust and wonder, need and sweet misery, love and grief—all the passionate derivatives of sex and death…" And there you have it. Original sin.

If I was going to deal with the art of being a physician, I wanted it all—science, medicine, pharmacology, surgery, behavioral things, human drama, existential questions, ethics—that's oncology. I, tongue in cheek, tell my patients that ever since I was a little kid, I wanted to be a breast medical oncologist—that I wanted to palpate (*feel* is a better word) breasts. They seem like better organs to study than the prostate, the rectum, or any of the gyn stuff. Certainly not the mouth or nose. I guess the heart and liver could have sufficed, but I chose breast medical oncology. An awful disease—breast cancer. A place where I too often see untimely deaths in young women, with too much time lost. I witness unrelieved pain and, the worst of it all, unnecessary suffering—all witnessed by my Jane. I remember one evening when I was reading in bed. It was a night when the kids had several of their friends over—all young teenage boys. Jane came into my room to tell me there was a wager going on about my work. I was curious. "What kind of wager?" I asked. They were trying to figure out the total number of breasts I had examined since medical school. They also wanted to know if it upset Jane that I had such an interesting job!

We, of all the living creatures, know we are mortal, that we are timebound and at some future moment will be no more. As Sartre says, we are "condemned to freedom." It is the ultimate recognition: not only I but everyone, everything I love and don't even care about, will be lost—today, tomorrow, in a forever limitless pervasive flow of reckoning. Yet, I must live my life, get up in the morning, work, pay taxes, feed the kids, and throw out the garbage. Living life daily requires me not to spend too much time thinking of inescapable ends, or I get nothing done. So what have I been looking for, if not the meaning or significance of my life? Some full worth to a truth of permanence—if not now, eternally? If not, is it all for naught—without meaning? I think, therefore I am, but worse—I thought, therefore I was. Somehow my consciousness is connected to my ability to participate in eternity—I lose self-awareness and I cease to be. How fragile this sense of life really is, as Emily Dickinson tells us: "Forever—is composed of nows."

> Below are lyrics from Bob Dylan's "Restless Farewell":
> Oh, a false clock tries to trick out my time
> To disgrace, distract, and bother me
> And the dirt of gossip blows into my face
> And the dust of rumors covers me.
> But if the arrow is straight
> And the point is slick
> It can pierce through dust no matter how thick.
> So I'll make my stand
> And remain as I am

And bid farewell and not give a damn.

There's no question that sometimes life seems so exemplary. It meets a standard that most of us cannot reach but that is always possible and attainable if we have the stuff to do it—Jesus may be out of range, but Gandhi and Martin Luther King Jr. and so many others could be models for a good life. And indeed, their life's worth and permanence are woven into the fabric of their deaths—a willingness to give up life for something noble, something larger than themselves. Are we obligated, if our lives are saved by someone or prolonged, to make certain we find a purpose for that extension? And we hope for them more permanence in an eternal blissful existence because we feel inside that goodness should be rewarded and evil punished. We would hope for Hitler to be rewarded not with an eternity of nothingness—a meaningless void—but with some type of retribution for his transgressions. I would hope that he would be given to all the dead Jews. Isn't this part of the kicker of my faith? The good should be rewarded and the bad should be punished in a heaven and hell?

Now we are getting somewhere—we need a deity to judge the good from the evil and claim ownership of judgment—all back to original sin and my grandmother. "Little Frankie, if you don't listen, you may end up dead in hell. Don't even think bad thoughts because someone is always listening and watching." My patients feel this. Isn't this what we want—some sense of retribution or reward, punishment or forgiveness—to make some sense of the deeds of a life? Doesn't that offer some reasoning for all this reality—value and meaning? Death, and all that it represents to those who believe in an afterlife, is the ultimate reason to live a good, moral life. In the *Phaedo* (63c), Socrates adds to this belief: "I am in hope that there is something for us in death, and as was claimed from old, something better for the good than there is for the bad."

And I wonder: Can my stream of consciousness—even more, my sense of self-awareness that makes me know myself—live on beyond death, in an afterlife, to accept the rewards of my life's deeds or the anguish of eternal pain? Eternity is a long, long time. The word doesn't really capture the idea of a self-aware being continuing on and on—not a thousand more years, but a million, billion, trillion years, on and on. It's hard to fathom, and is that what our dinky identities really want? Besides, I've changed in the reasonably brief time of my life here on earth. There is certainly continuity in my stream of consciousness despite the turnover of molecular change—I still identify myself as me and my memories as mine, although I do wonder if my memory of events, of people, is really the truth of how they happened or how I wish to recall them. I have said it happened that way for so long—is that the way it really happened, or was a dream meshed with reality? Now I'm confused.

We elaborate on the traditions and stability of what we believe is true so we can keep our identities and self-awareness, or it all begins to fall apart. Igor Stravinsky says of old age, "I wonder if memory is true, and I know that it cannot be, but one lives by memory nonetheless and not by truth." So here we are: we really can't spend too much time contemplating our dismal future—the whole of our cosmic doomed reality—and can't spend too much effort in believing our past is even authentic. I'm caught in the present—the now. Hopefully, this is authentic.

I am not certain I'm a more compassionate or empathetic physician since Jane died. Dying at home is a formidable endeavor—more than I had anticipated. It's a private affair, and maybe, in the end, it was better that it was just us two facing the end. She never wanted to seem so vulnerable, out of touch, not in control of the situation, and frightened about what was happening. I didn't feel much, except for hoping to cover all the bases—get her settled; make sure she was clean and comfortable, had no pain and less struggling. Now, looking back, I am amazed how little is said at a time of closure when everything should be laid out for exposure; there are only whispers of words tied to present insurmountable needs—a touch, a cool compress, a firm word to get her to rest.. No big struggles. No towering words of wisdom. No soft, comforting music. No solemn spoken prayers. No rosary. I feared the coming darkness of the night—to again be alone with her, wondering what was next or how hard this would get. Soon there would be no words. And again, her mantra, her forgiveness for me: "It's not your fault—this is not your fault." A gift for me.

PART VII:
Principles for Dying

I remember a medical student giving a definition of palliative care: "It relieves symptoms even if it kills you!" I know about this dilemma—it's part of philosophical oncology, calling on the principle of double effect. The rule of "double effect" goes back to Roman Catholic moral theological principles dating back to the Middle Ages. Christian thinking was clear—evil is neither inevitable nor an illusion but emanates out of the disobedience and rebellion in the Garden of Eden (Genesis 3:4) that caused mankind to "know good and evil." What this tradition tells us is that we humans live in a world where good and evil are cloudy, ambiguous, and often difficult to separate, and that we are called to be "cunning as serpents, yet harmless as doves" (Matthew 10:16).

The principle of double effect requires four conditions to be satisfied for an action to be permissible. First, the nature of the act must be good or neutral (e.g., giving opioids like morphine). Second, the intention of the agent (a physician, or in this case, me, the husband) must be to achieve the beneficial effects of the action (relief of pain and of shortness of breath).

Third, the bad effect must not be intended, but only foreseen and tolerated. The good effect must not be produced by the bad effect (relief of suffering must not be caused by death). In relieving the suffering, you cannot get rid of the sufferer. Fourth, the good that comes out of this—the consequence—must outweigh the bad effect. There thus must be proportionality between the good and bad effects. For example, relief from severe suffering can be achieved only at a high risk of death. In the end, obviously, this is not a legal formula but does serve as a moral guide for us to work with—even though the action chosen could lead to an end that would be seen as immoral if the end effect were directly intended.

It does make intention crucially important in moral reasoning, and criminal law is founded on a notion of motivation; common sense suggests that this is true. In 2003 I wrote a paper for the National Comprehensive Cancer Network discussing the principle of double effect in medicine. I remembered a paper in The Journal of Law and Medicine by Daniel Sulmasy , an American medical ethicist and former Franciscan friar. He wrote "Harms done intentionally are both bad and wrong…harms done unintentionally may be bad but in special situations, such as reckless negligence, are not considered wrong enough to be homicide." If I had decided to give Jane a bolus intravenous dose of potassium (assuming I was sound of mind) and had declared my motive clearly, the goal would have been admirable (to relieve pain), but the means chosen would not have been good (it would have led to unintentional killing).

One may argue that a person's intentions are private and unknowable. It may be, at times, difficult for a physician to separate personal intentions when suffering is severe and ongoing and the physician is without the ability to easily relieve the patient's pain and agony. The patient may be paralyzed from the neck down with inability to move, have severe shortness of breath, have intractable pain, be incontinent, and have severe depression and anxiety—all may lead the clinician to conclude that both intentions (comforting and hastening

As Good As It Gets

death) are not such terrible consequences. The physician may remain quiet, and the intentions may arise from a real sense of compassion but remain private and unknowable.

Some criticize the principle for having shortcomings as an ethical guide for the following reasons. First, the rule began within a specific narrow religious tradition. Second, current plural society calls for and often demands multiple traditions for end-of-life care. Third, the rule prohibits intentional killing, even if a competent dying patient asks for assistance. Fourth, individual intentions are hard to validate. Fifth, the rule has prohibited some confused physicians from giving opioids and pain relief for fear of blame. Nathan Cherny, a well-respected palliative care doctor, believes the justification for the use of sedation in the management of intractable, intolerable pain is best served by "goal appropriateness" and proportionality rather than the principle of double effect between the dose of opioids and the hastening of death. It may be that the risk factors considered clinically important to determine survival and impending death are not relevant in a study population only days away from death.

There is always a moral imperative for us as physicians to give medical care that comforts. As a husband, loved by and loving the person in need, all I wanted was to deliver care and all that implies. Nonabandonment is a medical philosophy that goes beyond the usual standards of legal negligence. My presence in looking after her and seeking attention to details was my gift of nonabandonment, with all the necessary elements of what care means: comfort, calmness, continuity, communication, and closure. In the final analysis, it is mercy and shared humanity that should win over any rules.

In the end, I had done my best. Despite feeling helpless, I had tried never to show my own anxiety and incompetence. This was a new arena for me—this was as close as it was ever going to get. I was a real, unadulterated novice, and I realized this didn't require IQ points or medical competency—it required being human to care for a loved one. Dying is hard, so I was never under the delusion that I could make everything go away, but I stayed present with constant vigilance. I listened as best I could to what was asked of me.

I don't remember exactly when it was, but on a late afternoon in 2006, I received a phone call in my medical school office. My secretary said it was the attorney general's office in New Orleans, but I had no idea why they were calling me. The American Society of Clinical Oncology (ASCO) had had its annual meeting in New Orleans recently, and I couldn't remember being that drunk when there. This would be the start of a different adventure in dealing with the standard medical care of patients at the end of life. Here, the advanced question was not so much about cancer or progressive disease but about elderly, frail individuals who needed the best of supportive care in unimaginable surroundings.

I was to become witness to an American tragedy. The attorney general's office had found and reached out to several sources who knew of my interest in the problems, questions, and ethics of people close to death. I wasn't expecting to deal with patients who were not known to be dying or terminally ill but who, nonetheless, were frail, with terrible chronic medical problems: history of stroke, diabetes, infirmities of old age, and morbid obesity, and incapable of being independent out of bed. Added to their frailties was the aftermath of a hurricane that had taken away the essentials of life—food, electricity, air-conditioning, water. This was a battered, struggling American city. I suggest that you read the story in Sheri Fink's *New York Times* bestseller *Five Days at Memorial* or in her *New York Times* piece "The Deadly Choices at Memorial," which won the 2010 Pulitzer Prize.

I was asked to review the charts of around a dozen patients who died about the same time with excessive amounts of morphine found in their bodies. Dr. Anna Marie Pou was at the heart of the story, a well-recognized head and neck cancer surgeon who had graduated from Louisiana State University School of Medicine. No doubt she had gone through the living hell of the hurricane. She was arrested for killing patients who were suffering the ravages of their illnesses, with death certainly a threat if they couldn't be moved. The Louisiana Department of Justice in Baton Rouge was filled with despair. There was no fervor to have her suffer anymore, and she was not indicted. I and other experts were not called to testify about what we had concluded in reviewing all the charts—that patients without terminal diagnoses but in a hell-like place were "put to sleep" to rid them of further suffering. This was active involuntary euthanasia. I wrote in my report that this was homicide, as did Dr. James Young, the former coroner of Ontario, Canada.

Were these acts of mercy that were trying to lessen suffering or acts of murder? The grand jury declined to indict Dr. Pou—and I can understand, despite my absolute conviction this was intentional mercy killing in an ungodly world created by God and man. John Francis Fink, newspaper editor and columnist writes about the biblical story of the wounded King Saul, who asks for death to end his pain: "Stand over me and kill me." The soldier who helped kill him later tells King David about his deed, and he is condemned to death. You tell me what is right here.

I read each of the dead patients' charts. The medical notes were succinct and often scanty in terms of real information. This was no clarity in the written documentation in those halls of hell, of despair and abandonment. The chart of Mr. Emmett Everett was the one that had the most impact on me. He was admitted with the problem of severe constipation. He was a morbidly obese Honduran-born man who was a paraplegic from a spinal cord accident. Emmett had no cancer or terminal prognosis except fate placing him unmovable in a bed that was also unmovable. His life ended there. I was seeing death again—unexpected, untimely, and painfully connected to the doctors who cared for the patients. Questions and more questions. What would I have done? I asked myself. I felt sympathetic to the physicians, and yet I felt something more could have been done to make them less culpable. This is a Shakespearean American tragedy that could happen again, since there is no will in our system to address the question without having to place blame and punishment. If there is no culpability, there is no fix for the problem if it happens again.

I have struggled with my final formulation here against these physicians, my argument that what I read about amounted to homicide. Was this catastrophic event really beyond my imagination or my ability even to make a rational judgment? These were not my timebound cancer patients running out of options but poor, vulnerable folks in unrecognizable normal life situations—and do the rules change? The ethical approaches need to be open and extended.

The physician must somehow offer to the patient the reasons and courage to make death a good death and, if nothing more, one with grace. Can there be a rational plan that is possible for a physician to undertake once the limits of medical objectives have been reached for any individual patient? The true meaning of reachable and comforting care arrives at that moment in time when there is a realization, if not acceptance, that the ravages of the disease cannot be made better. No one states it better than Paul Ramsey: "We cease doing what was once called for and begin to do precisely what is called for now." What is called for now, however, can be quite unnerving, weakening our determination and spirit of conviction because there really appears to be no one correct way to act. In these situations where we are facing life's ending, there often is the tendency to cover all bases, to act in the patient's best interests while respecting the individual's precious right of privacy and autonomy. We wish, obviously, to obey the laws enacted and follow our moral principles in any particular case, but we also continue to have deep-seated feelings about the action chosen. These innate emotional impressions can impair our logic in each case presented to us, even though we consider ourselves to be experienced, skilled, and concerned people involved in the necessary care of the dying. Precisely what is called for now is thinking clearly about what we are doing and examining the reasons that inform the actions we choose.

The spiritual nature of medicine teaches us to always accept the trade-offs of our care, especially when the alternatives are crappy. We often still hide ourselves in the complexity of our technology and machines when dealing with dying that is natural and inevitable. There is always something to be done for someone who is in pain and wants help. Medicine is not an unapplied profession but a moral activity and practice, one that is of the mind and hand and heart and intellect and character. What is called for, I have found, as a physician and the spouse of a dying wife, is unhurried and different—listening, positioning, comforting, cleaning, holding, touching. In the end, Arthur Dyck notes in an article in the *Harvard Magazine* (January 1976): "The moral question for us is not whether the suffering and the dying are persons, but whether we are the kind of persons who will care for them without doubting their worth."

The real criteria for limiting any treatment that prolongs dying must be based not on a life's "worthiness" but on our ability, as a free society, to recognize the difference between a human life's meaning and sanctity and an individual's or family's resistance to ongoing therapy at the point where tolerance of this protracted process of dying lacks further personal meaning. Our future horizon will be difficult when we attempt to decide on those cases in which the person exhibits minimal physical and cognitive function over extended periods of time. The procedural safeguards will need exploration for those persons who could not or did not leave clear instructions that define their sense of degradation of the life they now hold. What model of decision-making do we wish to have? I submit it should be structured on the assumption of clinical competency and advocacy, as well as with the patient's legitimate right of self-determination and autonomy in mind. It is a model built not on a physician's arrogance, professional codes of conduct, fear of medical liability, or irrational promises and expectations, but on mutual trust. I really believe that in the end, no court action, legislation, ethics committee advice, living will readings, or proxy statements will enhance the moral activity of medical practice if trust in the patient-family-physician triangle is truly dead.

I have been fortunate—no patient (or my spouse) has ever asked me to end their life because of progressive cancer or being terminally ill. Even better, I have never again found myself with someone so plagued by pain or misery as in Vietnam, where death was asked of me. I wonder what my conduct would have been toward those frail, vulnerable people trapped in the Gethsemane of New Orleans in 2005, after Katrina. I would have preferred that providence take hold—I believe that waiting would have been a better option, that there is and was a real moral difference between doing nothing at all and directly acting to take a life. If nothing else, I don't believe I could have withstood the lifetime of guilt for the deliberate act to bring on death, even, my God, if the patients begged me to hasten their deaths. Some moralists may disagree with me. I know of no case or prosecution of a physician in the United States for holding back care that would have extended life. My reluctance to kill would have been a paralysis, perhaps, of deciding, but that's fine with me, because it would have meant I was deliberating seriously regarding outcomes, needs, desires, and the rightness of the action. If nothing had been done to those poor souls, it would have been a diffuse decision among the caregivers, where no one would have been guilty of an act of killing. But again, I wasn't there.

In the fullness of unending time and immense geography, all known beings have ceased or will cease to be. We are condemned to this truth. We can ask, "Is this as good as it gets?" and just move on. Gottfried Wilhelm Leibniz, probably one of the smartest people ever around (the inventor of calculus) and a religious man, believed and wrote that God, who knows all and is all good, created a world that is the best of all worlds possible. In the seventeenth century, there were back-and-forth theological and philosophical arguments concerning this infinitely good deity—an all-powerful, all-knowing being who heads a theocratic world such as ours, filled with misery, suffering, and sin. Many have found this to be an argument against God's existence. Leibniz, however, believed that God is all-knowing, that He is aware, and that He can foresee everything over time. One of Dag Hammarskjold's notations in his book *Markings* suggests that only on a perfectly white tablecloth can one see a stain. And so here, too, "a little evil [can] render the good more discernible" and thus has a "permissive will," allowing sins to exist in this world. More to the point, this is what we've got—it is as good as it gets. As Steven Nadler, a philosopher, writes, this world is "metaphysically superior to all other possible worlds…one thing has more perfection than another if it has more reality." God has created a world that is "simplest in hypothesis, and the richest in phenomena," and it is here I dwell, and work, and will ultimately leave.

Let me return again to my grandmother telling me about the Garden of Eden story. That world seemed kind of perfect—even the animals spoke, or at least one snake did—and they wanted for nothing. I guess it wasn't as good as it seemed, because this is what we ultimately chose because of our free will. I really don't want to take this on, but one can write, and people have written, books about this story. I like to think I have free will, yet when I think back on decisions I made in the past, I do wonder: Am I the same person? What the hell was I thinking? In my defense, I guess, making a bad decision is not the same as making an illegal, criminal decision or an unethical choice. But a bad decision, such as not choosing the right mate in marriage, does have detrimental consequences—some of long standing. These consequences, in the end, affect other people—the parents, and more likely, the children, the residual product. And then, of course, they become the good consequence of the bad decision made in the first place.

I wonder, Do some decisions ultimately have to be made—whether we like it or not? So much for free will! Do we change enough to become different people? I think we do, but I also believe that that which is me, my day-to-day choices about a multitude of things, does create a person of character, one that is not perfect but at least acceptable—I know not to lie, steal, kill, talk unjustly about others. More importantly, I follow rules or do things not for the sake of avoiding hell but because I have hopefully become a reasonably virtuous human being.

The real trick is to navigate through life and medicine in those gray areas of life where there seem to be conflicting goods or competing principles (e.g., the patient's personal autonomy and the physician's beneficence toward the patient). Say that this action or decision is in your best interest (so providing it to you would be an act of beneficence). But you don't want it, for reasons that only you care about, so you don't receive it. That's called autonomy, where you have self-rule. Indeed, this can become a societal problem: we wish to protect the vulnerable, but there are obviously limited resources, and this scarcity of resources produces policies of limited and diminished beneficence. I guess it's worse to harm someone than to refuse to help someone. And then, who do we define as vulnerable—the homeless, the elderly? We are all familiar with the Good Samaritan story told to us by Jesus, so maybe I can be a Samaritan. Maybe there are no unjust policies, but there may be uncharitable and immoral ones.

Frank Sinatra quotes the comedian Joe E. Lewis as having said, "A friend in need is a pest." This is a cynical statement, but there is probably too much truth to it for it to be used as a political slogan of any party running for election. There are corollaries that seem to follow, unfortunately. First, the needs of the pest are usually the pest's fault. Second, the duty to help and give assistance is diminished at the extremes of the needs—hold the toilet paper; however, serve the meal. Third, the geographic proximity of the pest is directly related to the obligation to help. If you're in my face, it is hard to look away. In Africa, you're on your own. Fourth, it is easier to deny assistance to many pests than to one. That opposite always seemed like a good ethical rule—harm the fewest; deny the most. And finally, of all the pests' needs, the needs of the pest in the family are the worst to deny. Here you're on your own.

Medical ethics became an academic pursuit that grew out of medical technology dilemmas in the 1960s. Initially, there were real questions about who should be selected for hemodialysis. The first heart transplant was in 1969. Many patients were subjected to experimentation without their consent up until the 1970s. Minority groups were taken advantage of. At the same time, the cost of medical care skyrocketed, and a large population of our country lacked any ability to pay the rising cost. And out of all the amazing progress grew more complicated questions. Our country offered added conflicting issues: diversities of backgrounds, cultures, languages, religious beliefs. We have a long history of uniqueness, individualism, and geographical differences within our capacious borders, such as a more conservative, religious South and a more liberal, less religious Northwest. In the 1980s, there were a number of seminal papers and articles concerning ethical questions of assisted suicide and euthanasia. Jack Kevorkian, a pathologist, was prominent in the news for helping close to 130 people die. He was convicted of second degree murder. There were other seminal writers who wrote about medical ethical questions such as Eric Cassell, Timothy Quill, and Ed Pellegrino. Some states responded by relaxing guidelines and assisting dying patients with an easier end. It opened up questions for oncologists and medicine as a whole about our place and role in relieving pain and suffering, and now in the dying process itself. Hospice care was competing with this counterview that we couldn't always fulfill people's wishes to have an easier time with their illnesses. Indeed, what often was promised by technology and modern medicine could not be delivered. One great quote said it best: that we have become "gods before we are worthy of being men."

In many ways, trust in our fellow man has been lost, and we've become cynical, sarcastic, depressed by it all—sometimes all on the same day. We dislike lawyers, and we have too many running the show—including in the federal and state governments, hospitals, and television commercials. And yet the law, as a whole, always seems to be on the side of protecting the patient against the government's abuse of power, as evidenced by disagreements among numerous parties on numerous topics—for example, informed consent, human experiments, and emergency treatment. It is important to follow how final legal decisions are formulated. Look at the minority view that's held: "If the sheep and wolf are to vote on the next meal, I want to know how the sheep thinks." I like that one.

In a specific medical situation, Frank Brescia should or should not—the ought question—do something based on what? Principles? Values? Whose values? Law? Or the consequences of his actions or inaction? There are well-known, described principles to follow. First, autonomy, which stands for an individual's self-rule and self-determination. Man is an end in himself, with intrinsic value. Second, beneficence, or best interest, as the patient as a person sees it. Third, the counterpoint: nonbeneficence. Simply put: do no harm. And finally, justice, which means treating people fairly and with equality.

Aristotle taught us that moral reasoning involves applying these general principles and skills to specific situations. I, as a physician, a medical oncologist, become a moral agent for my patients. My decisions in caring for them have profound implications, especially for those most in need, most vulnerable, and perhaps the most hopeless, whose true medical care has become futile. My decision-making is usually based on a long-held belief in the intrinsic value and sanctity of life, compared with the obvious counterpoint that there can be a time and situation where life's value is diminished and nonabsolute, as defined by the patient, loved ones, the facts, and the reality of advanced, progressive, fatal disease. I must find understanding in empathy—what I would want for myself—and compassion for the patient.

The person I usually treat is complicated. Aren't we all? Just look around at your family and friends. People, indeed, have conflicting needs and sicknesses. Above all, illness steals away from us the ability to do or be what we want—it is a "thief of autonomy." More to the point, patients' needs and concerns are often altered and not articulated or communicated because of their distress, depression, and fears. One can ask correctly, "Is the real person speaking?" Is it authentic, even if autonomous? It may be very difficult for the physician to process correctly or understand what patients need, how they view the world now, and what they ultimately want. It's even worse when they no longer can speak for themselves.

Thank goodness I have had very few requests over the years from patients requesting that I help them die. "Doctor, I want to die. Will you help me?" Even my Jane, in all her distress, especially at the end with such air hunger, never even came close. I'm so glad that request was never made of me—how much more grief and anxiety could I bear? I thought she might or could ask, but she never did. In surveys published regarding physicians' attitudes and beliefs toward the legalization of euthanasia and assisted suicide, the results from the past are interesting. Diane Meir published a national survey in the *New England Journal of Medicine* that found the following: Among 3,102 physicians across ten different specialties, 11 percent would hasten death with a prescription that they would write. Seven percent would give a lethal injection—this number I thought was low. Of note, 4.7 percent said they had given a lethal injection, and 16 percent had given a prescription to aid. Slightly less than 20 percent of patients had made a request for aid in dying—certainly a much larger number than I ever had. In another report in *JAMA*, 355 randomly selected oncologists in the United States were surveyed: 16 percent reported having helped a patient die, 2 percent had performed euthanasia only, 28 percent had performed assisted suicide only, and 8 percent had done both.

I've thought about this question of aiding death a lot since my Jane's death. Pro arguments are quite reasonable, and I can empathize more now: it is a sincere form of love, care, and compassion for a small group of people with intolerable suffering as they define it for themselves. Certainly, this gives these people a sense of control—something they have lost, some of them for a long, long time. And they are tired of life. It does prevent botched suicide attempts and all that musters up. Some would say this is really a last resort and most often a seemingly rational decision. Is it a personal right of choice?

The law is mixed. Surveys seem to show popular support even though this option is not often requested or accomplished.

Counterarguments are also strong: killing via euthanasia is always morally wrong and goes against medicine's mandate to heal and do no harm. We already talked about the difference in the principle of double effect. The concern has always been that implementing euthanasia as public policy will lead down the slippery slope to broaden the category of people suffering: handicapped children, the elderly, the poorly responsive.

Our law ultimately chooses and legislates the morality of the society we live in. Law, though related to ethical guidelines, develops from our societal customs, our community's reflective values. The law mediates between what appears to be right from different sides; it ultimately makes compromises and mediates between the opposing views. While ethics can be described as an inquiry of principles and rules, of examining the consequences of actions, the legal system ultimately enforces the morality of a society—whether it's with laws regarding when and if abortion can take place or laws about whether I can help a terminally ill patient die. The law finally tells me—it mandates some action, or inaction, and there is no longer time for debating. The ethical controversy and considerations continue.

Left to their own whims, patients will, from time to time, choose to die on their own time, when and where they choose. Will they always make the right choice? Certainly, the decision represents a dramatic, democratic point, if not the high point of their lives. Would my Jane have gone directly to hell if she had ended her life?

Life, to these individuals, is just not worth going on with—there's too much of a price. Are the decisions made with real, authentic critical reflection, on the basis of personal desires, not pushed by other people but thought about over and over and over again? Here's the ultimate query: Can our government prohibit and prevent people from choosing assisted suicide or euthanasia? Even more crucial—believe me—is the question each one of us needs to ask ourselves: What would you do for a loved one who asked you to help them die? For my part, I would have to realize there is a sufficient, unavoidable reason to help someone die—a case would need to be made to change my overwhelming reluctance to help kill someone. I see only potential harms if helping people die becomes a broad social policy: Will we always have consent? Can assisted suicide or euthanasia be forced on vulnerable people? Will we absolutely try to help those with mental illness and depression? What about children? Are we certain we have the best, and I mean the best, of medical and supportive care?

I think our principles will survive—and we physicians will always need to apply them to specific clinical patient situations and see if they work for us. Every ethical theory thrown at us, I suspect, will have flaws. In the end, I must go back to remembering that I am a moral agent for my patients, that maybe I should ask the questions in ways that are virtue based and not just through guidelines. This also requires a virtuous community with values—always related to a healing doctor-patient relationship.

Some clinical situations, I think, are very clear—we know what we should do. An example is the story at Memorial Hospital in New Orleans in 2005 following Hurricane Katrina. As I've described, patients were suffering the ravages of an inhumane and seemingly hopeless situation when apparent relief was given with morphine and Versed. Yes, again, in getting rid of the suffering, we get rid of the sufferer—this is a scenario where there is not a school in which to find character but a test of character. But here, the community—society—saw this collection of acts as acceptable. Society did not condone these actions but said, "Let's give the moral agents a pass."

No doubt, just as there are clear clinical situations in which we know what's expected of us physicians, there are more dubious ones where, again, the left side of our brain tells the right side to take a nap. We must always mediate through the phenomenon of sickness and all it represents to persons and the goals of medicine and healing. I don't know how else to say it. There does seem to be meaningless suffering—we see it all about us, and we want to help rid our world of it. Particularly, I want to alleviate (a) the untimely deaths in my young breast cancer patients, who are no longer able to live their lives or watch their children grow, (b) the sickness of children, (c) the decay and decline of aging, and (d) pain and distress, especially in our ignorance as to why we must suffer these things.

PART VIII:
Suffering: A Test of Character

Why did Jane have to suffer? Now we come to the hard questions about life, illness, and God. Ah, and isn't the unnecessary, undeserved suffering of the innocent an argument against an all-knowing, all-loving, all-merciful deity? As an oncologist, seeing tragedy upon tragedy, I know that one can become cold to the totality of calamity on any one day, and the only way out is to deliver doctoring at its best. This is what compassion means—what bioethicist Edmund Pellegrino has described as the character trait that ultimately "shapes the cognitive aspect of healing to hit the unique predicament of this patient." Meanwhile, for the patient, "Hope dwells in this dimension of existence, and great suffering attends the loss of hope," as Eric Cassell tells us.

It is unnerving to see what the cosmos can throw out at us to stalk and menace us, for us to endure. Many of my patients with a diagnosis of curable breast cancer spend a lifetime anxiously waiting for the sky to fall upon them. We do seek some control of our lives and mercy and forgiveness in the end. The unrecognized beauty of concentrating totally on little-noticed details of our lives is lost completely when serious illness, raw abandonment, and death surround our being. The daily drama of life becomes too heavy and burdensome, and all the details seem unimportant, as summed up nicely by Alice Trillin, a young teacher with lung cancer:

> One of the ways that all of us avoid thinking about death is by concentrating on the details of our daily lives…they become a burden—too much trouble to think about. This is the real meaning of depression: feeling weighed down by the concrete, unable to make an effort to move objects around by ennui…we think too much about our bodies, and our bodies become too concrete—machines not functioning properly.

I was a young physician just out of my oncology fellowship at MSKCC in the mid- to late 1970s. It was one of my first consultations as a young attending. "Please see this man with newly diagnosed malignant melanoma" was the request—a devastating diagnosis during that time, with minimal treatment options beyond surgery. It was not quite fifty years ago, but still this man's story haunts me with the devastating calamity that he lived through; yet it also gives me, in some way, a sense of hope in how we live—as trite as all that may sound—and what we bring to the table, the stuff that holds the human family together, our shared humanity.

I'll call him Mortimer. Mortimer was an accountant with a personality and demeanor that fit the role. He was an anxious but extremely talkative man with a need to know the slightest of details about everything—pathology, day-to-day care, lab work, next steps, everything. He was married to a woman with a British accent and, as I remember, had a son in law school. Sometime in the 1950s, Mortimer had fallen off a home ladder trying to repair something on his roof—he broke his neck and became a quadriplegic, and the only appendage that could move was his thumb. However, he worked every day, had an attendant that helped care for him, and managed to get the most out of moving his finger. Why was I seeing him? He had recently been diagnosed with a melanoma under the nail bed of the only moving digit—that thumb. Treatment was amputation, strike one. Within the next two to three years, he developed metastatic disease and ultimately brain metastasis with confusion, headache, and further neurologic deficits. I remember, in the early days of caring for Mortimer, deciding whether he would be the first patient of my rounds or whether I would save him for last.

It was never an easy visit—because of his illness, my inability to make things better, his personality, and the obvious pain and suffering and loss he was experiencing. His wife visited daily—never upset, always composed, well dressed, and put together. I never saw her speak harshly to staff or appear frustrated with the terrible experiences she was living. Mortimer suffered severe progression of his brain metastasis and obviously was dying. While that was happening, his bright, sole child, who was in law school, collapsed and had a massive cerebral hemorrhage—I forget why. AV malformation or brain aneurysm. Mother and wife would visit both her son and her dying husband. One night, late, I saw her at the hospital elevator, going home, and I had to go up to her and ask, "How do you do this? How do you have the necessary energy even to get up?" Her answer was quiet, simple, and given, as I remember, with grace and poise. "We lived a good life. We always told each other how much we cared for and loved each other. I believe there is a reason for everything that happens to us and that tomorrow will be better. I believe God will explain it."

I've thought about this a lot over the years. I've read Eric Cassell's pivotal writings and Ed Pellegrino's insightful philosophical thinking about illness, suffering, and medicine's role—particularly the doctoring of us physicians. I realized this in caring for my wife, Jane, and during my own bouts of threats to my health and life. The person we see as a patient assumes a new role and status that is unique and special, separating him or her from all who are seen as well and healthy. The person becomes a patient when the illness strikes and some lived, personal experiences of the self can no longer tolerate and bear, alone, some real or imagined complaint or need. Each of us has a different threshold in terms of what that is—sometimes the distress is also compounded by fear, denial, or a history of witnessing the same in a loved one.

We can also ask this question: How must we view the specialness of each of us—view personhood (self) in a time of great advances in medicine and technology, with the traditional Western philosophy of dualism separating and splitting the mind from the body? The body can be objectively observed, studied, examined, and literally dissected by hand or by modern machines—CT scans, functional MRIs, PET scans, and so on. Descartes insisted that man's nature consisted of soul and body, each a complete substance. He postulated that the soul worked in a particular place in the body—the pineal gland—but he had great difficulty explaining how the body (a material substance) influenced the soul through any causal link. The scholastic, traditional explanation of body and soul complementing each other as one complete substance, therefore, was neglected.

Eric Cassell, a practicing clinician in New York, philosopher and author wrote often about the role of medicine in treating suffering: "Cartesian Dualism made it possible for science to escape the control of the church by assigning the noncorporeal spiritual realm to the church, leaving the physical world as the domain of science. In that religious age, 'person,' synonymous with 'mind,' was necessarily off limits to science."

We don't understand how consciousness and self-awareness work, but the question remains: Is it all material—my brain—or is the brain a receiver of a universal and fundamental consciousness that is cosmic and currently unexplainable? In the end, the subject of my consciousness tears into the question of an afterlife and non-timebound existence—and perhaps a deity.

We are, necessarily, confronted with the issue of the permanently unconscious being, which is suggested by some to be devoid of any human dignity and personhood. Some would suggest that personhood and autonomy require consciousness, while others see thought only as a physiological, anatomical, and complex biochemical reaction.

In a chapter called "Body and Self" in *The Humanity of the Ill,* Sally Gadow writes, "The body becomes the concrete otherness of the self for itself." The body becomes what is known to be potentially and eventually vulnerable to the entire landscape of disease and injury. We do live our entire lives always ready from birth to face inevitable natural evils—sickness, disability, pain, and death. The body cannot distance itself from the self. The equilibrium of the body-self is broken when the indignity of illness causes the body to become an impediment to the experienced living self.

Lloyd Bailey's great description is worth reading from his 1979 book *Biblical Perspectives on Death:*

> The human dilemma is that we are caught between two worlds, the one symbolic and the other animal: we are able to transcend nature and speculate about the mysteries of the universe—able to experience awe and love, able to create value systems—and yet we are part of a body that aches, stinks, and dies. We are able to soar, physically as well as mentally, among the stars, yet are destined to rot beneath the ground. We are beautiful of form, yet constrained to bodily functions that shame us: "gods with anuses."

Again, Eric Cassell emphasized the necessity for medicine to address the patient as a person, with all that implies and gives, while avoiding the traditional assigning of the body to medicine and the person (self) to the category of mind. He concluded that if, indeed, we accept this dichotomy as valid, suffering is subjective only, and *not* in modern medicine's domain. This thinking depersonalizes the sick and becomes a real source for delivering more unnecessary suffering.

Thinking about this is important because suffering occurs to all of us in time, with differences only in kind, timing, and degree. The sick person "chooses" the intimate reasons for his or her own pain, for there is ownership of and propriety for this anguish, which no other person can truly understand because it's not being experienced. It must be lived. It dominates self-consciousness, causing, as Louis Lavelle tells us in his book *Evil and Suffering*, an "interior agony in which the self acquires in this very suffering it experiences an extraordinary lively awareness of itself." The person thus becomes a stranger to himself. "Who I am" no longer exists in the same way. "Who I am," not "who I was," or "who I want to be," or "who I ought to be." The beauty of being human seems to rest in our ability to find meaning and value in the most severe reduction of what it is to be healthy and whole. Mortimer and his wife taught me that lesson: I am not the generic universal patient—I am me.

We do learn from each other in both the good and happy times as well as the bad. We live singular lives, but we do not live alone. There is no history, no future, apart from engagement with others. Again, Cassel says it wonderfully: "No person exists without others. There is no consciousness without consciousness of others, no speaker without a hearer... Take away others, remove sight or hearing, and the person is diminished." And yet suffering remains totally personal. Who will share meaning with me?

Doctors know too often suffering exists, but because they feel helpless and impotent to do anything about it, they ignore it. By not being present to this calling out, they may add to the anguish of their patients. For example, when I prescribe chemotherapy to a young woman with breast cancer, I may be doing this to reduce the statistical risk of recurrence. If I choose one of my better drugs, paclitaxel, because of its statistical benefit, I must also be aware of potential short- and long-term adverse side effects such as sensory peripheral neuropathy—which may cause constant pain, burning, tingling and fine motor damage. If my patient is a violinist or painter, and I take away her beloved talents, she now has both the cancer and her loss of function and identity to think about. I've made her suffering worse. The need to listen is even more critical and important if the patient is actively dying. The hope should not be to get more toxic drugs but to be with family, to be supported, to be loved. The hope is not to travel—it's to see the doctor and get blood work if little more can be realized.

It was this past week when I saw a returning patient who raised what Bart Ehrman, a professor of religious studies at the University of North Carolina, describes as "God's problem." The patient has a history of an aggressive form of breast cancer that required intensive multidisciplinary treatment—surgery, chemotherapy, and radiation, as well as hormone-blocking medication. None of this comes without residual end points—fatigue, neuropathy, cosmetic alterations, and potential heart muscle damage. No longer working, she has, at least for now, no evidence of recurrent cancer—and that is good. Her husband of over forty years recently died of lung cancer after a difficult course of treatment, and my patient carries a great deal of anger toward his oncology medical team. She weeps each visit talking about his loss and final days. Her nearly forty-year-old son recently died of a fentanyl overdose—he was found unresponsive in his bed. She sobs again when she talks about her son. But then she quavers, "God is good. There are reasons we cannot know why things like this happen."

I say to myself again, I wish I had this kind of faith in the God whom I was taught to love and whom this woman believes in, the God who is all-good, all-knowing, and all-powerful. Again, I have to first believe in a God before I can be angry with Him. I have to commit to the notion that this is the best possible of all worlds and that God permits evil to exist. The Jesus of my Catholic faith died on the cross for the stain of the original sin of Adam and Eve—for all of us. And in this act, he does not remove the problem of human suffering, but indeed, as God incarnate, the second person of the Holy Trinity, the one God, he partakes in the suffering of the crucifixion.

Epicurus (341–271 BCE), as quoted in Steven Nadler's book *The Best of All Possible Worlds*, puts the problem in easy language to understand: "God either wishes to take away evils and he cannot, or he can, and does not wish to, or he neither wishes to nor is able, or he both wishes to and is able…

If he neither wishes to nor is able, then he is both envious and weak and therefore no god. If he both wishes to and is able to, which alone is fitting to God, whence, then, are there evils and why does he not remove them?"

There in a nutshell is the conundrum: God is all-powerful, all-knowing, and all-merciful, and bad stuff still happens to good people. Evil exists. Maybe there is no evil. Maybe evil is, as Robert Nozick terms it, a "privation." I love this theodicy explanation: as with Aquinas, the theologians agree that "evil is nothing real and positive in ontological terms; it is the negation or lack of good." Tell that to the person with a knife sticking out of them from a robber! Thus, we can define evil as an imperfection of the created reality—not perfect. And with this God-created reality, we have suffering and physical calamity and moral evil and sin. Why in God's name would God do this and choose this reality? The explanation from Leibniz, who was, mind you, one of the smartest persons to ever live, is this: because of God's perfect goodness he created the best world possible, allowing permission for free will. And thus he breathed life of existence into this best possible universe, which is "metaphysically superior to all possible worlds." This world has the maximum capacity for perfection over all others because God, by being God and perfect, could see all the other possibilities. In the end, "God wills antecedently the good and consequently the best." Stanley Hauerwas, Professor at the Divinity School at Duke University would say the suffering should be not a school for character but a test of character. I like that better.

I do so want to believe in God. But at the same time, I don't want to delude myself. I listen to and read arguments for and against the possibility of God, and my head turns. Some pro arguments are too nuts even to consider, but they are here. For example, this is Saint Anselm's thinking regarding God's necessary being: "Therefore, if that, than which nothing greater can be conceived, exists in the understanding alone, the very being, than which nothing greater can be conceived, is one, than which a greater can be conceived. But obviously this is impossible. Hence, there is no doubt that there exists a being, than which nothing greater can be conceived, and it exists both in the understanding and in reality." Did you get it?

Aquinas talks about the desire for perfect goodness to exist, and as a cause it is prior to being. Got that? Then there's the ontological argument—if it is possible to have omnipotence and conceive of such, it must as part of its essence be actual existence. OK, I'm lost too!

I think I am more inclined to consider the idea of purpose behind our history of cosmic birth. These are magnificent equations, so fine-tuned, within incredible narrow limits, that allow our place in the sun to exist and allow me to be. This is known as the anthropic principle—where only this fine-tuned place we live in could allow us to come to fruition, and in it are all the physical laws and equations to give us the opportunity to behave.

Here there are purpose and divine design. I do want to believe. But the atheist says we don't need God's existence for all this to happen, and indeed we could have come from nothing on the basis of the laws of quantum mechanics, or this ultimate reality never had a beginning but has always been. I give up! I surrender. I still must deal with my patients' suffering and their (and my) questioning. Why?

I go back to reading Job. Not only is it a literary marvel, but it is also telling us about this ultimate human problem of the why of suffering. Edmund Pellegrino, a physician-philosopher, wrote of Job specifically for physicians to think seriously about in their work. Jonas Salk often wrote that in science, it's not the answers to findings that are important but always the asking of the right questions. We get no answers from Job, but the questions it raises teach us about ourselves and force us to ask how we will respond when faced with iniquities.

We cannot escape the shared human experience with Job. For me as a physician, he is my patient. For me as a person and patient, Job ultimately is me. Can I respond with such patience and really believe good can come from evil? More to the point, am I satisfied with God's seeming indifference and apathy to my hurt? Can I not turn against this God of flagrant indifference to my loss, sickness, and suffering? Paul Claudel, a French poet-diplomat, called it "the most offensive book of the Bible." In the end, Job explains to us the terribly personal experience suffering brings to us—each of us—along with, in the end, a test of our humanity, the thief of all our autonomy. Job fails to give us answers from God, and we damn well know God will not answer us.

The "Why me?" question has always been a thorn in my side. My mother, a deeply religious woman, could not understand how a diagnosis of pancreatic cancer could fall upon her. Was it some form of punishment for some unknown sin? The Latin root of the word "pain" is *poena*—this word also relates to punishment. Isn't this the basis of the oldest story in the Old Testament? Job suffers ranges of loss, calamity, and illness—he is a righteous man, but he is criticized by his closest friends and told that he must have done something to deserve all this punishment. Oncologists hear this at the time of a patient's diagnosis, at the time of recurrence, and at the time of progression and approaching death. David P. Steensma, a professor at Mayo Clinic, says it well: "Blaming the victim is a very old pastime." Things can be bad enough because of the disease—add to it the sufferer's belief that something he or she did caused this impediment. Guilt and anxiety are thus added to whatever is going on physically—a double whammy. And one wonders if this undeserved agony is redemptive—does it bring any good, and to whom? It's hard to recognize any good in the suffering of ill children, who must feel the toxic effects of chemotherapy without any understanding of the why.

God, I guess, answers Job's question with a question: Who the hell are you to even ask such a question? Where were you when the cosmos—this universe—was created? And your "friends" who scorn you are also wrong! How that tale enlightens us to see it as it is—there is no answer that makes any sense to me. And when we are with those suffering, we should just stay, "Settle in, be present, and be *silent*." And we move on to the next.

PART IX:
Random Reflections — Trying to Pull It Together

So here we are, we mortals, looking out at the edge of the vast ocean and sitting on a fragile pier where the end is absurdly uncertain and immense. The size of the mystery of reality presents such unimaginable truths that we are ultimately unable to comprehend what there even is to comprehend. As the comedian Lewis Black says, "The right side of the brain tells the left side to take a nap."

The Hubble Space Telescope was given a simple chore: look at a small patch of space as it made four hundred rotations. It found in this minute patch of geography ten thousand galaxies, each with billions of stars, some of these thousands and millions and millions of light-years away—a light-year representing six trillion miles. That is far and big. And all we want is a little love, health, happiness, and maybe some closeness to each other.

What's my place in all this—my contribution to this cosmic mystery? Especially since I also have to die and never find out what it was all about in the first place. My Catholic upbringing always told me that the reason I'm here—the purpose of my existence—is to be with God, and particularly with the resurrected Jesus. And boy, do I want to believe that it's true—that God is real, that He lives somehow in some realm, and that not only will I have myself to continue endlessly with all my memories, but I will also see those I so yearn to see again, all those I've loved deeply. And I look, so as not to be deceived, for all the reasons and arguments about why there is a God and all the counterarguments that there is no plausible reason or need for God's existence. I go back and forth: On the one hand, I tell myself evolution is the divine design and the cosmic presence looking at itself. On the other hand, I wonder if we are just randomly chosen to be here by some natural physical law. If so, a divinity is not required. But if a divinity is present, where does that entity begin? Can there be a cause without a cause for itself? And why? The concern I have with my Catholic faith has always been the incredible amount of arrogance regarding knowing the "truth" absolutely—the absurdity of that indisputable certitude.

It seems, however, that believing in something is important for most of us, especially those with critical illnesses or at the end of their lives. Harold Koenig, Professor of Psychiatry at Duke University Medical Center and others in 1998 looked at 542 patients and their psychological and social well-being. Nearly 90 percent felt that having faith and religious beliefs was important to them. Indeed, 60 percent participated in daily religious activities. Gerard Silvestri, at my institution, the Medical University of South Carolina (MUSC), examined one hundred advanced lung cancer patients looking for help in making decisions about their treatment. All patients ranked God second after their medical oncologists for help in decision-making. Highly religious individuals are three times more likely than nonbelievers to receive intensive life-prolonging treatment near death and are less likely to see hospice care.

Often, patients will reflect on being abandoned by God—that no prayers are answered. Some of my patients are quite silent about what really is going on in their heads. I think half my dying patients are seeking some forgiveness for something or from someone. This certainly is the right time. I must admit that near and at the end, conversations become limited—patients struggle for the next breath of life or strength to keep their eyes open. Often religiosity is now replaced by a more spiritual tone focused on the nature and world around us. God is missing and nowhere to be found—it's an atheistic spirituality. But this too can become an amorphous, flawed, and empty endeavor. To quote Samuel Butler, "To be dead is to be unable to understand that one is alive."

Personally, I'm not good at religious ritual activities. If I am going to pray, it will be alone—or with my piano. Let me praise the Lord in my own quiet and confused way. Once at the oncology clinic, quite early in the day, I noticed the medical and nursing teams had their heads down and quietly were praying. Indeed, they started each morning with this small ritual. I had given no opinion to them—and to be sure, I really did not have any to give. One morning, the lead physician, a woman, along with the nurses, walked over to my side and asked nicely if I wished to join them in prayer. No question—if I turned them away, I would be a heathen. Yet I really did not want this to be forced on me—a perpetual opening-day prayer. I had to think fast. I suggested the following: I *would* join their prayer vigil on one condition—and we *all* had to agree. Each morning I would spell out a list of names, and we all would pray that each one would have a miserable, lonely death. There was gentle chuckling—crazy Brescia—and I was disinvited from the group. Sometimes, I think I am not a good person.

And then there was Anna, ninety-plus years old, admitted with intestinal obstruction related to her known GI malignancy. Frail, weak, wasted, but clear and very much with the matter at hand. "No NG suction tube for me," she stated emphatically. Surgery? To try to relieve the obstruction? Again, she was as clear as one can be: "There are only two people I want to see—my husband, dead some years now, and Jesus, my God." Can't argue with that kind of faith and honesty of resolve. No one was changing her mind and tune. Oh, how I wish I could be that strong in my convictions—it would make it so much easier. Maybe that's the conversation that those doctors should have had with the patients after Hurricane Katrina. "What do you want us to do? Give us some guidance. We can't get you out, and you're suffering terribly now, with little hope of getting through this—help me know what to do." Maybe that's a conversation too hard to endure, with an impossible response. Again, I wasn't there.

We seem to crave immortality, a going on indefinitely, not wanting to get off this drama-filled stage. Someone needs to get a large hook to snatch us off. I'm always amazed at my most religious patients, who are always talking to their personal friend Jesus and who seem to have the most trouble, wanting to get to see him—wanting that faith healer and miracle. They would have placed a feeding tube in Jesus on the cross to extend the suffering. As Woody Allen tells us, "We don't know what to do on a rainy Saturday afternoon."

I don't know what the limits of time should be on our lives—a proper life span. Nozick writes, "How unwilling someone is to die should depend, I think, upon what he has left undone, and also upon his remaining capacity to do things." Regrets fade as we become less capable of doing things. It seems we would perhaps be better off with the eternity and immortality offered by death and an afterlife—whatever that state of existence may consist of. An envisioned immortality of continued earthly life may be a sustained condition of tedium, sameness, weariness, tiredness, and dullness. No reason to ever take something seriously—a kind of oblivion more perhaps like death, always the same.

There is, it seems, a certain nobility and dignity to mortality. As Carlos Castaneda noted in *Journey to Ixtlan*: "Decisions of an immortal man can be canceled, regretted, or doubted…In a world where death is the hunter, there is no time for regrets or doubts, there is only time for decisions." Hell indeed may be the enchanted geography where you have your way forever. We can't escape from the inescapable actuality of our lives, and we are not going to get any help from God, the cosmos, our earth, the devil himself, or fate. Death really is the most democratic of events—a dramatic change for us—and because we must all die alone, our dependency on one another makes each singular death intensely shared. In the end, the confusion for us is why the cosmos gives permission for our deprivation of all the things and people we most care about. Hell has been called truth seen too late!

If we concentrate on a mental picture of the experience of being dead, we quickly get lost in language, fears, visions of an experience, or religious reflection. Epicurus is the most succinct, "If we are, death is not; if death is, we are not." Right away we see the problem: there is no experience to connect with. We can't conceive of the phenomenological experience of being dead. We have no experience! What has no limits of space and time can't offer an experience. We are left without change and remain unmoved.

There are questions concerning death that fall into religious or philosophical traditions. One: Is there complete extinction;-we cease to be? Dust to dust. Two: Is there continual rebirth—as something else? We turn to seed to be reborn as fruit. Reborn as whom? I cannot even guess. And in what temporal realm? Do I get time off, or if time is an illusion, can I come back in the past? My past? Three: Do I somehow keep my conscious self—my personality and memories? Do I preserve my free will? Four: Can there be a higher state of reality and melding of other conscious souls or God? Do I finally understand reality and the truth of what it's all about? Do I see those I loved? And five: Is there something else I cannot even ever realize? I suspect this may be the most likely.

We come to know death through the continual loss of others. There is this constant train of loss and grief, and the human connectedness that we have to our families and others is forever irreversibly broken by death. This interconnectedness of our lives is very fragile, and we again are left alone. Past, present, and tomorrow are eventually all gone. And I'm looking for some point to this narrative. Why death? Wrong question. Why life? As noted better by others, "As soon as birth, one can be ready to die, and death doesn't rob life's meaning but makes life's meaningfulness possible." This is spoken by Death himself in the classic 1939 film *Death Takes a Holiday*.

We are just renting this space and time, like in that expensive watch advertisement. Mortality awakens our ignorance about everything—about the answers to the questions I've been pondering and especially about a deity who I so badly want to believe is real, both for me and for everyone I've ever loved deeply. We are all so afraid of this darkness of understanding regarding God and all that follows. Julian Barnes, in the wonderful book *Nothing to Be Frightened About*, suggests for us to go on and believe; it does no harm. More to the point: a nonexistent God will protect you from nonexistent elves and demons. Montague, a great essayist, gave us the first modern thought regarding death: "Philosopher, c'est apprendre à mourir" (*To philosophize, is to learn how to die*).

So God does seem to have a crucial role in my thinking about death and dying. It's important for my timebound patients to know how to frame their own illness and decision-making. Trust the doctor—trust in God more. To some of us, it's thinking of God less as the creator but more as the arbiter of judgment of past misdeeds and transgressions. We seem to think there needs to be an accounting, and do we indeed make the grade? If I'm sick and dying, my God, somehow, some way, will show mercy and save me. But he must exist and be real. One may wonder, seriously, if God is OK with an honest doubter, perhaps like doubting Thomas. I guess if you really believe and have faith, and God does exist, you should get some credit for this. However, some are not so assured because the justice delivered out in this world doesn't give us hope that we'll see it in the afterlife. Will there be free will in the next life?

We don't want nothingness—no reason to have been, with no grief or remorse left behind. I want someone, or many people, to have cared I existed and grieve my absence. That's why it's important for God to exist—because He should, I hope, care. The universe is alarmingly silent and unfeeling. It doesn't need my existence to continue—and indeed, it is better without me to take nutrients and space from the newcomers. My despair is in seeing my demise from the vantage of all the strangers who never spoke to me, heard of me, or cared if I ever lived—an unknown, unnecessary obituary. The surgeon Sherwin B. Nuland writes that billions have died for us to live—to keep a state of balance. Even worse, Camus tells us, "We are beings without a reason for being." We are the stuff of the reality of the universe, and never should we forget that we are intertwined, not separate. I must create meaning for my existence. And the question remains: Why do we need a God to care for us?

And yet there is something very special about us individually—the number of genetically distinct entities is one followed by ten thousand zeroes, meaning the genetic possibility of the humans who have been created is less than 0.00000...000001 with 9,979 added zeroes—this is noted by Jim Holt's treatise on why there is something rather than nothing. Around forty to one hundred billion people have already existed. As he describes it, "I exist—a beacon of certitude." The ultimate point is that I do exist, and maybe I shouldn't care there is no meaning, value, or purpose. It goes back to Job's question and God's answer—Don't even ask the question, you little shit. Wow! I am special. Holt describes it correctly: "My improbable existence has a curious counterpoint—I now have to imagine my nonexistence." Interestingly, the fact of my nonexistence before my life doesn't relieve me of the future terror of nonexistence. You've got this—you've done this already. Someone said we want perpetual peace, whatever the hell that is—perhaps it means having just enough life to have enjoyment in being dead. Is it terrifying to not be born? Jerome Groopman tells us about his patient Kirk Bains in *The Measure of Our Days*: "See if you still find that enough comfort when you're the one in this bed. Nothingness. No time, no place, no form. I don't ask for heaven. I'd take hell, just to be."

That's what we would define as a singularity—outside space and time.

I love Schopenhauer—the Woody Allen of philosophy. He takes our fate to the dark side, noting that our being, our existence, must be a kind of mistake—an error. "It is bad today, and every day, it will get worse, until the worst of all happens." Sounds like he would be fun at family gatherings.

Did I gain wisdom? This human desire to survive death—is it because I want some larger task to allow me to find a larger purpose than myself? But what is that, and how long does it take to get there? I'm well aware of my limitations, and I wonder if this is as good as it gets—I need to do more. I'm fearful of the incompleteness of my life, of what I say to those around me, of what I leave behind, the loss of being loved and loving. And love is so crucial to making our lives better, giving them worth and meaning—yet always we know in the backs of our minds that it's going to end. Either we go first or they go first. Again, that's why religiosity soothes me—I may see these I loved so again.

Consider the obituary that reads "He is survived by his wife of fifty years of marriage." I thought no one survived death—even the dead person really is not a dead person but represents the remains of someone who was once alive.

I really shouldn't take these errors of language too seriously—they are not going to change and most likely will get worse as time passes. I cannot wait for the next morgue sign—let's see how hospitals can defrock the word "morgue" even more. Once, a long time ago, I received a call from a nurse about one of my patients in the hospital who was known to be quite near the end. The nurse started by stating that the patient did not look well, that she could feel no pulse, get no blood pressure, and hear no heartbeat with her stethoscope. Then she waited for me to say something, I think. A pause. And I asked quite simply, without anger or sarcasm, "Is he dead?" A longer pause: "I think so." It is such an overwhelming, awesome conclusion. I guess I should have understood better. But nonetheless, no "decedent affairs" next—just death.

And yet, with all our fretting and denial of it, it does surround our world. Both historically and daily. Just read any newspaper every day. There is an obituary about somebody—not us, but somebody. Sometimes we read about large numbers dying over short time spans. For example, thirty million died from the plague over a five-year period in the 1300s. Thirty million died in the 1918 flu pandemic over the course of one year. Then 2,753 were lost on 9/11 in just two hours. And even more alarming, seventy thousand died at Hiroshima in 1945 in just five seconds! Astounding! There are dormitories of resting space we all pass. When I lived in the Bronx, I would drive through the Woodlawn Cemetery, opened in 1863, with its over four hundred acres of fertile land holding over 310,000 souls—some quite prominent, like Herman Melville and Duke Ellington. My grandparents are buried there.

The American experience is interesting. Fewer than 1 percent of us die annually—the changing of the guard, the flushing of the population. But we do live a bit longer than our grandparents. In 1900, the life expectancy was forty-nine, with the majority of all deaths in children under fifteen attributed to infectious diseases. Now, a woman of seventy-five can expect to live another twelve to fifteen years, and I see more and more patients over one hundred years old. Roughly 6 percent of people with Medicare coverage die annually.

I must admit to my own demons of denial about what's happening to me. Ashamed as I am to confess, these sins are quite real, and they show, without any question, how much Jane was right—I am an idiot. I really can't answer the why of it all—just attest to the fact of either denial or stupidity. In 2005, we took my adopted daughter Joy back to China—visited her orphanage and planned to see multiple sites in her country of birth. This would be a three-week discovery for me of a very large and interesting country—more so now that I had an adopted little girl gifted to me by some of its people. We made a deal with my daughter that she would prepare a talk about this visit to China, charge a donation to hear her talk, and give the money to her orphanage. Joy raised over

$2,000 before we left, and indeed, we gave some of the money to the orphanage, and we used some to buy toys and needed supplies its staff requested. Everybody won—and my daughter needed to pay attention to describe what the trip meant to her. I was proud of what she eventually did when we got back home.

Several days into the trip, we visited the Great Wall. It was summer and quite hot. I had become more fatigued with each day, but this walk on the wall was noticeably more difficult. I had no history of any significant illness but had a strong family history of cardiovascular disease—my father's first heart attack was at age forty-five, and he died at age sixty. He was, to be sure, overweight, he never exercised, and he ate what he liked—all not good—and he had been a two-to-three-pack-a-day Camel smoker up until his first heart attack. His father—my grandfather Frank—died suddenly at age sixty-four, a smoker at the time. My uncle Leo, my father's brother, died at thirty-nine—same story. I knew the history, but I never smoked, was not overweight, and ate, perhaps, a little better than my father. But on this hot, hot afternoon on the Great Wall, I was struggling with tiredness—no pain or shortness of breath, but I was not able to keep up with Jane, which should have been notice to me that something was not quite right. I told Jane I had to stop. "Go on ahead of me—I'll sit," I said. And I did. I recovered but remained tired for the rest of the trip.

At home, I began to note new, progressive discomfort within my shoulder and upper back. We had been working vigorously on our house, moving furniture and throwing a large amount of old and unused stuff out. More pain, more with movement, and relief with stopping. At times the pain was severe enough to stop me in my tracks. Motrin (not a good idea) seemed to help—in fact, I had a twenty-four-hour pain-free day. I claimed I had beat this. Only the pain came back the following day with a vengeance—now severe—and I needed not show this to Jane. The night before admission to the hospital, I had this vivid, towering, epic dream. I was at the cemetery—a mausoleum of my family. We needed to move somebody to get somebody new in. I had a blocked left anterior descending vessel and needed a stent and medication, and I got a scolding from everyone. That happened seventeen years ago. Dumbass!

In 2016, we had a family trip to France planned with my wife, seven kids, my sister-in-law and brother-in-law, and my wife's parents. We would spend three weeks in Normandy and Paris and take a cruise to Budapest. Four days before our flight, I had routine dental cleaning done—no big event. Ten days into the trip, I started to feel ill with fever, chills, fatigue, and a mild cough. No big deal—just a bug, I thought. My mother-in-law had similar complaints. She recovered, but I did not. By the end of the "vacation," I was having a nightly 102-to-104-degree temperature, rigor and shaking chills lasting forty-five or fifty minutes, loss of appetite, and cough with some pleuritic-like chest pain. Should we see a doctor here? No, of course not. The trip home was hard, with me being pushed in a wheelchair by my ninety-year-old in-laws. What the hell is wrong with you? I thought. My ultimate diagnosis after a week home was sepsis from the dental organism *Pepto streptococcus*—this organism is exquisitely sensitive to penicillin, which I was given intravenously for six weeks! Dumbass. Strike two.

My recent stupidity again showed a flair for absurd denial and medical incompetence. COVID had struck, and I needed to work at home—a good thing, except I wasn't feeling well. This came on quickly over a few days—maybe a week. I became really tired, but I had difficulty with sleep because I needed to pee often, three to four times per night. Then I also had to pee more frequently in the day—seemed like every thirty minutes. Thirsty. Give me anything—water, chocolate milk, orange juice, beer, more water. My tongue was wooden, dry. Pictures on walls seemed to take on animation-like characteristics. My wife and daughter seemed nervous about me. I suffered a vivid hallucination of a strange woman wearing this bluish-green feathery 1950s outfit coming to bed with me. I didn't recognize her, so I told no one about her. Strange. I was having trouble with the order of words—saying things like "melon water." Thinking was harder to do. So thirsty. Blood sugar 1,300+. I was admitted to the medical ICU with two lines of fluid going in. A1c was fourteen or some obscene number. The severity of the high blood sugar was strange and a surprise since I never had a diagnosis of Diabetes. With exercise, some dieting, and time it resolved. No more insulin needed. I was better and back to work.

  Why the apathy? Why the denial? Is it because I'm a physician, or a man, or just fucking stupid and in denial, or all the above? Have I learned my lesson here? I know I can't do this again. My family was mad at me. I was mad at me. I could see how quickly someone could get into trouble alone, avoiding the obvious—this is not normal. This is not a prostate thing. We got a problem here that needs some attention: polyuria, polydipsia, fatigue, dry skin, blurry vision. Good thing you have someone who cares for you, dumbass. I think I'm wiser. We'll see.

PART X:
New Life: It Begins Again

Soon before my Jane was initially diagnosed with breast cancer in June 2004, I had an interesting patient, Suzanne, diagnosed with a very similar breast cancer with nearly the same stage and biology. They both had a two-centimeter tumor, with Jane having a micrometastasis in one node (less than two millimeters), and my patient with negative nodes. Suzanne went on to chemotherapy to prevent recurrence with two terribly nausea-producing drugs: Adriamycin—affectionately called the "red devil"—and cyclophosphamide. Four doses were given every three weeks at that time. Suzanne not only sailed through treatment but also seemed to thrive, playing three or four hours of tennis at the nadir of the chemotherapy cycle. I couldn't believe it. Suzanne was in her late forties, a tall, really stunning, and athletic woman—a Katharine Hepburn type. She was married, lived in Hong Kong, and was diagnosed with breast cancer while visiting her parents here in Kiawah, South Carolina.

After Jane's diagnosis, I tried to prepare her for the chemotherapy side effects and noted how well this one patient had done. I knew Jane's journey would not be as easy—she had terrible nausea and vomiting with her pregnancy, a potential guide to who is going to have a problem with chemotherapy. And by God, I was right. There seemed to be no end to the nausea, awful metallic taste, vomiting, and weight loss. She swore she could not continue—but she did, and it eventually came to an end. She said, "I need to meet with this woman—this patient of yours who doesn't throw up with this. I must meet her." How and when that meeting occurred I cannot recall—all I know is that it did. They became the best of friends, talking into the night because of the time difference between South Carolina and Hong Kong. Suzanne would let Jane stay in her New York apartment when Jane needed to see doctors in New York. Every detail of their lives seemed to have been shared. I've never been quite sure that Suzanne's doctor—namely me—was not shared as an imbecile, but the story moves on. One never knows the twists in one's life story.

After Jane's death, I was comfortable with being alone—in fact, I remember a particular Sunday when I watched football at home alone in my underwear, thinking, "This isn't so bad—I can do this. No running orders." I was surprised by the close friends who offered one of their woman friends as a potential date—even a judge—even an Italian American judge. I declined. I thought I really needed a life pause. It was just me and the dogs, who, by the way, made the journey bearable during that period. The fall and coolness of winter came. Life went on. Notes to friends, work to do. Calls from my kids. I was renting a home—indeed, I had sold everything. There was no permanence here. I recommend that feeling of freedom for everyone, even if only for a short time.

There are events in our lives that seem inconsequential, banal, unimportant—that are open only to retrospection, that are to assume monumental importance later in life. A chance meeting, an awkward glance, a kind word—all seemingly fleeting moments that come back to haunt the future. An introduction of common ties somehow can alter the future interconnecting of lives. For me, such a moment occurred when I met Suzanne's older sister, Christie, at one of Suzanne's appointments—she asked reasonable questions about Suzanne's care. Occasionally, when Suzanne would visit, there was Christie, also coming to meet with Jane—who always had some advice for anybody about anything. Christie was married with two children and was often with her parents in Kiawah.

After Jane's death, Suzanne asked her sister to occasionally see how I was doing. She brought flowers for Jane's memorial service. Then several weeks, perhaps months later, we ran into each other at the hospital where she volunteered. Pleasantries were followed by an innocent hug, and we were on our way. That evening, she texted me to see if I wanted to go for coffee. I learned she was now divorced and living alone not too distant from me. Here's where it went downtown. I suggested we have dinner at Cuoco Pazzo ("Crazy Chef"), we set a date for a few weeks later, and bingo—we were off to the races! We talked that cold evening—we were the last to leave the restaurant, with me thinking that this was really nice. Maybe two months later, a second dinner, then a movie and a third encounter. The following spring, I had thought about a trip to Paris alone—however, Christie had a history of going to high school in Paris, spoke French, and was willing to be my guest come spring to Paris. We were married on January 23, 2016, at her parents' home, with no kids crowding the place—no way to easily get all eight together in one room in mid-January. If not eight, none. Good choice.

And yet, love again—different, but no less meaningful or satisfying. The music and symphony play again with joyful notes, and I don't want it to stop. I ask myself, How is this possible? No answer. It is as real an experience as before, with the same sense of concern, affection, and bonding that I remember from before. God forbid I lose her, I think. Could I withstand again the daily ritual of facing future grief? It would be different, but the same. I suspect that, in the end, Christie and I would do our best.

Life moves in a straight line, always forward. Did I make this decision, or was it made for me? It is scary to retrace all your steps back to find out where you are now. As Yogi Berra said, "When you come to the fork in the road, take it." There can be happy decisions that only later, in retrospect, tell me there was a happy ending. If there is someone or something to thank for my fortunate finding, then I now declare my thanks. I would have been OK alone—it would have been a simpler existence. But as in music, a single note can be striking alone, but a chord, particularly if it has sharps and flats attached, is much more enriching, giving the listener a reward of sound. One rarely is awoken, alone, smiling—now I smile because of these symphonies of chords—some sharp, rarely flat or off key. One can only hope two lives are enough to create a symphony with a subtle beginning, interesting middle, and dramatic, satisfying ending. One can only hope.

I still work, fifty years out from my medical oncology fellowship. I think my patients like me not to retire and Christie likes me not home as much—so this is a good partnership. I joke maybe I'll go until I'm either incoherent or incontinent—whichever comes first. But being around younger, more energetic physicians and nurses fuels purpose, forces me to engage, to see purpose in always learning something new, and tells me I have something important still to offer. Even more, I carry history with me—of what it was like to make $5800 annually, see an unlimited number of admissions, work every other night, and be chronically tired but needed. This, I believed, was what made a physician special and gave the profession a noble calling—the person was a patient, not a "client," and death was not a "negative patient outcome." How could I tell my superior faculty attending that I was tired at 10:00 p.m. on the hospital floor when the faculty attending was there along with me? I felt part of something greater than myself, and always special—a good doctor who would not and could not abandon the patient who was assigned to be under my care. Everyone knew what we sacrificed in time, relationships, money, and pain. It was hard, but because it was hard, it truly was worth something. And I think I'm also afraid to stop working because when I do, that which is me, Doctor Brescia, is no longer the clinician, healer, or physician. It's tough to give that sense of who you are away—to transfer that torch. Maybe they need to get the hook to snatch me off the stage. Dumbass. Maybe?

So here I am. This has been an attempt to reflect on the major issues I've faced as a physician—certainly not exhaustive of the multitude of medical, ethical, social, spiritual, and psychological problems I've encountered. But that wasn't the point of this meditation, which is really more for me than for anyone reading this.

Let's recap—I've lived, I think, a colorful and interesting life. Maybe I *will* work until I'm incoherent or incontinent, whichever comes first. I still feel competent, empathetic, respected, and with purpose. I'm OK once I get in the vertical position from the horizontal and tell my wife next to me, "I really don't want to get up and go to work." It is amazing what standing up, showering, and having coffee does to change one's mind and attitude. I walk no fewer than three times per week and often five to six times each week, usually with my attorney daughter, Monica, whom I would have killed when she was a teenager if there were no laws against murder. I play the piano—not classically well, but well enough to make people think I'm at least acceptable. I'm not a jock. I hate golf, I never fished, and I never played tennis—I was more of a stickball person from the Bronx, and it's hard to gather anyone nowadays to play. I like to read about philosophy, and I must confess I hate books about death and dying.

I'm married now to Christie—she never changed her last name, and I can't blame her. Her upbringing was totally alien from mine—no curse words were spoken, and food was not the first thought of the day. She says she loves me, and I believe her, finding that as her only major fault. She is smart and world traveled, speaks fluent Parisian French, and is incredibly good looking and sexy for a woman in her seventh decade. Her parents are in their nineties—the father is nearly ninety-six, and he played tennis into his early nineties. Bob graduated from the Naval Academy, flew fighter jets, and retired as a colonel in the marines. His sister, as of this writing, lives at 102, and their father died at the freaking old age of 107. They've accepted me into the family. Their other daughter is Suzanne, who befriended Jane and introduced me to her sister, Christie. Life's circles are scary.

My regrets are bothersome and haunting at times. I don't think I'm alone:
- Married too young at the age of twenty-three. Why didn't they stop me?!
- Married the wrong person too young—divorced and annulled
- Should have stayed at MSKCC after my fellowship
- Turned down chief residency at MSKCC to go into practice in New Jersey. I wanted to start making money.
- Met Jane in 1983 but did not pursue a relationship at the time. Just stupid!
- Married briefly too soon after divorce
- Did not spend as much time as I should have with my kids when they were young
- Never learned Italian
- Never really learned to play the piano really well
- Did not tell those I loved how much I loved them

But there have been lots of good things, too:
- All my children: A, F, MA, M, M, J
- My family
- My time at Fordham
- My time at MSKCC
- Vietnam for making me a better man
- Beverly
- My MA in philosophy at Fordham for allowing me time to read and think clearly
- My life with Jane
- My life with Christie

As Good As It Gets

- Purchase of my Yamaha piano
- My move to Charleston, South Carolina
- Incredibly good friends: PG, SK, PB, JF, TC, JG
- Good doctors I have known
- My patients—all of whom taught me something about life and love

Peter Schjeldahl, in a wonderful *New Yorker* piece (December 23, 2019), concludes, "Human minds are the universe's only instrument for reflecting on itself. The fact of our existence suggests a cosmic approval of it…we may be accidents of matter and energy, but we can't help circling back to the sense of meaning…" He also suggests, "Take death for a walk in your minds, folks. Either you'll be glad you did or, keeling over suddenly, you won't be out anything."

I enjoy happy endings. Can I see this for myself and those I love and have loved? And what, you may ask, does that really mean? I want to understand this ultimate immense reality of which I am part. I want the cosmologists, the philosophers, and the theologians to discover and come to an agreement regarding that question. Michio Kaku, in his book *The God Equation,* ends with, "If we find the answer to that, it would be ultimate triumph of human reason—for then we would know the mind of God."

Nearly thirty years ago, on February 14, 1990, NASA's Voyager 1 spacecraft sent home to us a picture in sixty photos of our family solar system—a portrait of who we are. This was delivered to us from 3.7 billion miles (6 billion kilometers) beyond our sun and way beyond Neptune. We are a sesame seed in this photo. If one sees us as we really are, one can have an epiphany, a realization of our singular, vast insignificance in this inexplicable cosmos. Maybe my vast insignificance is the reason for the vast indifference and apathy of the universe. After reviewing these pictures, I shouldn't worry about my demise, my puny existence, any longer. The only absolute certitude here is my awareness of my existence and presence—my necessity of being present in this immense, cyclopean mystery of awe in space and time. I scream inside that I want to have mattered—I long to believe that somehow my existence caused a difference that would not have been if I had not come into being. Is that too much to ask for? And more, I am bound to the whole legacy of others who came before me, whose awareness and questioning are just like mine. I am looking for meaning. Evidence that somehow my life mattered.

Thomas Lynch in his book *On Metaphor and Mortality*, plays it well: "The facts of life and death remain the same. We love and die, we love and grieve, we breed and disappear. And between these existential gravities, we search for meaning, save our memories, leave a record for those who will remember us."

We can't think about this stuff constantly, or we will sit in some corner and never do anything again—but at the same time, we should occasionally address what, in the end, is the most fundamental wonder: us and our existence and ultimate fate. We can think about our parents, if not ourselves, regarding the stakes of the losses that occur during the process of dying. First, we see the decline of our physical health and our ability to do stuff we like to do, and finally we have to have someone do the basics for us—keeping us clean and well groomed. I know that I will lose my role as a provider, my worth, my status as the decision-maker of my family. Eventually I will lose them—spouse, children, possessions. Probably the biggest loss is that of a future—something we all need—and finally I will lose hope that tomorrow will be better than today. And then I will need to see if there is a loss of my relationship to God—if I believe and have real faith that my consciousness survives. Do I lose meaning as a being with marked significance and nobility?

I am trying to discern what has given me the most joy and happiness in and for my life as a whole—the rewards of my place here on earth. I'm looking inside myself to find the true richness of my whole remembered reality—the awe of recognizing what was true worth and value to me. Thomas Nagel suggests that "part of the problem is that some of us have an incurable tendency to take ourselves seriously. We want to matter to ourselves from the outside." He concludes with the thought that "if we can't help taking ourselves so seriously, perhaps we just have to put up with being ridiculous. Life may be not only meaningless but absurd."

I didn't die from my heart attack at age sixty-three in 2005. A bout with bacterial sepsis after a routine dental cleaning didn't get me. Even my superlative blood sugar of nearly 1,400, along with a few hallucinations, failed to end my run. So I ask myself again: Having lived past these failed attempts on my life, have I added time to a meaningful life? I love some of Robert Nozick's explanations of a potentially meaningful life. He gives the following examples. First, a "full productive life." We'll check this one off. Second, "the meaning of life is love." His take on this is probably as you see it—boring. However, there are other takes on this theme. Third, my Catholic religion tells me the meaning of life is to be nearer to God—ultimately with Him in the afterlife. Why doesn't this make me feel better? Fourth, an eternal void -this certainly, really doesn't help me. Nothing is bad enough. Eternal nothingness really doesn't satisfy my hankering for meaning. Fifth, death itself gives meaning to life. This is Viktor Frankl's conclusion. I understand how this works, a little.

I'm asking for the absurd, aren't I? I'm asking too much, and I should go on with my life, in fact, I'll go take that nap, wake up, and think about something else. Maybe I should remember God's answer to Job's lament and realize that no answers are ever given, so don't even ask the questions. Just have faith and trust, and it will all come to you soon enough, whether you have faith or not. I'm starting to consider that the mystery of my existence, the physics of the universe, the beauty of how human consciousness allows me to smell coffee in the morning, the immense size of the geography I live in—all these are way beyond even my understanding. Everything I can imagine—all the possibilities, and I mean everything—is on the table as possible. If there is any certainty about anything, there it is—certitude that anything is possible. Where religious beliefs fail us, I guess philosophical explanations can take over. Unlike in science, where asking the right questions is crucial, there is no help here—the question remains always open. There is an immense mystery regarding why I'm here and what the ultimate place is, if there even is any—the question is a mystery. There is absolutely no phenomenological experience I can fall back upon for answers about the mystery of ultimate reality, external existence beyond earthly life, and the meaning of this immense geography and journey.

My self-awareness—my consciousness—gives me, in this existence, the ability to look inward and ask the question about meaning because, without it, nothing really would make any difference. Consciousness becomes the fundamental tool to reflect on what this ultimate reality really is. We know by our conscious awareness about the knowing, and that we are the ones doing the knowing—how cool is that? Descartes said it well: "I think, therefore I am." We can add, "I thought, therefore I was." Pierre Teilhard de Chardin, a Jesuit priest, in his book *The Phenomenon of Man*, tells us that man discovers that he is nothing more than evolution becoming conscious of itself. I don't care about small individual pieces and select parts of the mystery, or the complicated mathematical equations—I want to comprehend the whole thing and understand how I, in my small and short existence (if there is no afterlife), fit into the picture. Disturbing is the absurdity of it all, if, as they suggest, it all collapses on itself and disappears. This sort of ruins the majesty and significance of it all, even if it goes kaput tomorrow or a billion billion years from now. Why? And do I really want to live forever? Longevity comes to an end. "Death keeps no calendar," noted George Herbert in 1640.

I have the same existential anxiety as the next person. I, too, have asked these same universal queries regarding the why of suffering in the world, and pain, and sickness, and raw evil. The death of us all seems to be the reason to open up the questioning about everything. I consider my insignificant self, who was born suddenly between the eternal bleakness—the nothingness of the past—and the scary possibility of going right back to the eternal bleakness, the nothingness in the future. I don't seem concerned that I once didn't exist, before my birth on February 24, 1942, but I do mind the necessity of ceasing to be. There is an asymmetry to our timeboundness.

And yes, I want to be remembered and to have mattered. It's been said, sadly, that we are truly dead—*truly dead*—when our names are no longer mentioned or spoken again. How long will that take? Not long, I suspect. When, indeed, the grave sites have no more mourners and visitors—that to me is true sadness and emptiness. We cease to be, collectively. But as Thomas Lynch writes, the dead may not care—they are at peace, but they matter. The hearse always leads the parade of cars. We pay tribute to the hyphen between the years shown to us on the tombstone.

As a physician, I have often seen the patient as a person at a time of vulnerability and weakness—not as the person truly is. Indeed, patients never reveal their true selves. Often, it's the times when the patient is seen with loved ones when you realize the connectedness of our lives and what each of us means to another through love. You can witness the place of that life and its significance to others. I observe.

Sometimes I wonder what is worse, my regrets about my past—the incompleteness argument—or the possibility of my not being able to see something happen tomorrow. Jane sobbed when dying, not for any life regrets but for her incapacity to see us grow old together, to see her children blossom, to witness her children's children. We can be cheated of life's most precious gift of experiencing—we fail to really live. Fredric March takes on the persona of Death in the 1939 movie *Death Takes a Holiday* and ponders why we humans avoid him—and discovers that *because* we ignore his presence, we miss the magnificence of life.

Is there any unity and wholeness and fullness that can be explained in one's life? Life has been pictured as if we are at the end of a dock with the unknown, vast ocean before us. Do we want to place our feet in the water and get them wet?

But I must confess to you that I am in awe of the mystery before us and all that's hidden from me—the immensity and majesty of the mystery. I really am special—I was born and came into being with numeric odds and genetic possibilities against me. I am a rare possibility, having won the lottery, rare among all possibilities—and yet here I am, and with me come my children, my grandchildren, and their children. I've come to be among a community of others—maybe seventy to one hundred billion others—with a history dating back millions of years, during which we acquired consciousness, awareness, language, tools, spirituality, the concept of a higher being, and above all, the curiosity to question everything about everything. I have seen the beauty of a woman's form, experienced the music of Mozart, Beethoven, Gershwin, and Cole Porter, listened to Sinatra, Tony Bennett, and the Beatles, and marveled at Michelangelo and da Vinci.

I will die, like my grandparents, my parents, my children, and my grandchildren's children. But we were all here, where we observed and took our places around the table and looked both inward and to the mysteries of distant stars. We shared all the gifts that existence gave us to enjoy and experience. It was meaningful for me to be, to care, to love, to touch, and to share the breath of life.

PART XI:
What's Next?

At some point in the near future, I will stop doctoring and give up my white coat and stethoscope. *Abbastanza per oggi!* Enough for today! My fifty-plus years will be enough, and I will move on, taking off the persona of the noble physician—yet still be me. I must, as we all must, retire. I'd like to think of it as being reborn. But am I fooling myself? Should I see this as a retreat, a giving up of this faded white coat that I have become? This new form of me will be free—finally free of the requirements of accountability, responsibility, and keeping up to date with the knowledge of whatever the hell I am, at a minimum, supposed to know. That initial reversal of me occurred long ago, when I walked into the cadaver lab as a young man. It was to change me from part of the laity to a professional physician with specialized knowledge. I will soon change teams again and join the masses of people who are witnesses to what medicine and doctors can and will do tomorrow. I will be relieved of hours of study about the most novel procedures or newest medications. No longer will it be necessary for me to attend national scientific meetings to hear what's happening.

And best of all, I will be free of the duty to respond to family members for every sneeze, cough, blistering rash, minor pain, or discharge.

I will lose, eventually, my network of physician referrals, and I suspect I will lose the badge of being one of them. Will I cease to be seen as someone with wisdom, someone deserving respect? There will be no more calls from drug representatives to offer me information about their new exciting drug or their need to give me a pen as a gift. I will miss the aura of being the physician-teacher, the one who knows the answer to the problem. Will my presence be missed by my patients, those whom I've touched, examined, and cared for? I know so much about their hidden stories. What will I do with all the time I once needed to solve all those mysterious ailments and confusing presentations? How fast will my reversal take, and will I no longer care about being the good and noble physician?

My mind and brain have been wired for so long to think in terms of reducing bodily stress and offering advice. They will need rebooting. I often wonder now how I am perceived as the older clinician in the room. No matter how well or exceptional I feel, I still compare the old photograph of myself in my office with my current image in the morning bathroom mirror. I notice the change and the mismatch. I remember so well that after my fellowship, patients acknowledged my youthful appearance, which translated into my look of lack of experience. Now, I am worn down from the burden of experience, and I now look the part of the near-retiring physician. Sometimes, I wonder if my patients suspect their next six-month or annual checkup will bring them a new and younger physician. I must confess I now think more about how I am perceived by my peers, nurses, and patients. Am I a liability or a blessing? I'm needed because I'm needed, but when there comes a time when I'm needed less, I may be seen as an incommodity. Will I be a drawback to have around?

Sports figures always talk about going out at the top of their game. I think often about it in those terms. I must keep up with the stuff. I must pay attention to details. It must never seem old or same-same, but always fresh, with each case and problem created just for me to solve. I must never be cranky. You have heard and seen it all before? The truth is that even now, after all this time, it is always different, challenging, amusing, and always testing my experience, talents, and skills. I must not be the best physician of the year, but I must always, each year, be the most improved. I don't want to miss something or deny someone ever because of tedium and tiredness. I would then know it was time to hang the white coat up. I'm spared the problem of the surgeon who needs both physical and mental endurance to sustain a long career. I have only to think clearly and keep my wits about me.

And then there is the new retired life at home. My poor wife, Christie, will have to face me, for better or worse, for longer hours. I will have to accept a new married role, and she will have to tolerate my constant presence. Can love that survived beautifully with me not around all the time be sturdy enough to survive with me there all the time? That will be the test. Will I be painting snow scenes with pheasants on the walls of the house like my father did? Can we hold hands with affection rather than with the fear that if we let go, we'll kill each other?

I accept that I will lose my specialness. After all, there is praise that I get from my work and from the staff that will all disappear, and I will be the retired man, unpraised around the house. That may be the biggest hell for both of us. We will need to talk openly about this new lifeboat we're living in and the change that will take place with my rickety self constantly roaming about the house. I, and especially Christie, will be in tremulous fear of what I may become and bring home. I may descend home with the infectious virus of despair of a new, purposeless life. Somehow, we must both work out a contract for each other to be mutually needed. And then love will be reinforced with purpose and satisfaction. I do not want to miss being what I was.

I will gain the wonderfully treasured gift of time by doing absolutely nothing. The ability to do only what I wish to do at any moment. I want to be free to smell the coffee and play the piano in my underwear. That is as good as it gets.

I've thought seriously about the what-ifs of my life as much as the "what was" and the "what is" of my life. One can replay the origins of one's life over and over, all with different outcomes—some better perhaps and some worse perhaps. I have had one singular life and have remembered it in my stream of consciousness through various shadows and memory. It could have turned out quite unlike what happened. The United States' entry into the Second World War could have been avoided if the Japanese hadn't bombed Pearl Harbor. My birth might not have been necessary as a contingency to keep my father out of the war. I could have not married my first wife, or I could have run off with Beverly in Vietnam or gotten killed in the war, whether married or not. There could have been no children that I raised, none of their offspring born, and suddenly the world would be remarkably different. If I had courted Jane as I should have in 1983, she might not have had her accident, or her child, and we might or might not have had our own biological kids. My adopted daughter from China would be in China. My piano playing might have been more worthy of praise and attention, and I might never have become the physician I became. All my patients would have traveled a different path of care. If I had not gone down a hallway to get a prescription at lunchtime, would I have missed love again with Christie?

So again, I ask myself…I was here and lived the life I lived, with all the stains and bruising of misdeeds and regrets. Was it a worthy life with value, meaning, and purpose? And who can better answer that question than I? Would any of the infinite number of lives that could have been, other than mine, been as worthy? If I really could go back, knowing who I am now and what I know now, would I change what I've done or become? In the end, I ask myself: Have I achieved happiness with a joyful existence, and am I satisfied that this was the best that it could have been and no better? In the end, it was better than I ever thought it could be. It was as good as it gets.

FURTHER READINGS

Alda, Arlene. *Just Kids from the Bronx*. New York. Henry Holt & Company, 2015.

Bailey, Lloyd R. *Biblical Perspectives on Death*. Fortress Press, 1979.

Balboni, Michael J. *Spirituality and religion within the culture of medicine*. Oxford University Press, 2017.

Barnard, David. *The epistemology of medical care*. Medical Humanities Review, July 1992.

Barnes, Julian. *Levels of Life*. New York. Knopf, 2013.

Barnes, Julian. *Nothing to be frightened of.* New York. Knopf, 2008.

Barnes, Julian. *The Sense of an Ending*. Vintage Books, 2011.

Beauchamp, Tom L. and Perlin, Seymour. *Ethical Issues in Death and Dying*. Prentice Hall, 1978.

Brescia, Frank J. *Philosophical Oncology, Calling on the Principle of Double Effect*. JNCCN Vol. 1, pp. 429-434, 2003.

Cassell, Eric J. *The Nature of Suffering*. Oxford University Press, 1991.

Cassell, Eric. *The Nature of Clinical Medicine*. Oxford University Press, 2015.

Chalmers, David J. *Reality*. Norton, 2022.

Chalmers, David J. *The Character of Consciousness*. Oxford University Press, 2010.

Christakis, Nicholas A. *Death Foretold*, Prophecy and Prognosis in Medical Care. University of Chicago Press, 1999.

de Botton, Alain. *The consolation of philosophy*. Pantheon Books, 2000.

de Chardin, Teilhard. *The phenomenon of man*. Harper Tourchbooks, 1959.

Ducasse, CJ. *The belief in a life after death*. Charles C. Thomas, 1974.

Duffin, Jacalyn. *Medical Miracles*. Oxford University Press, 2009.

Ehrman, Bart D. *God's problem*. Harper One, 2008.

Ferry, Luc. *On love*. Polity Press, 2013.

Fink, Sherri. *Five Days at Memorial*. Broadway Books, 2013.

Frankl, Victor E. *Man's Search for Meaning*. Simon & Schuster, 1959.

Gawande, Atul. *Being Mortal*. Metropolitan Books, Henry Holt & Company, 2014.

Glasser, Ronald. *365 Days in Vietnam, The Forgotten Hero*. G. Braziller, 1971.

Grealy, Lucy. *Autobiography of Face*. Harper Perennial, 1994.

Greene, Brian. *Until the end of time*. Knopf, 2020.

Hauerwas, Stanley. *Suffering presence*. University of Notre Dame Press, 1986.

Hick, John H. *Death and eternal life*. Harper and Row, 1976.

Holt, Jim. *Why does the world exist?* Liveright Publishing Corporation, 2012.

Hyde, Micheal J. *Perfection*. Baylor University Press, 2010.

Institute of Medicine. *Dying in America*. National Academies Press, 2015.

Johnston, Mark. *Surviving Death*. Princeton University Press, 2010.

Kass, Leon R. *Toward a more natural science*. Free Press, 1985.

Katz, J. *The Silent World of Doctor and Patient*. Free Press, 1984.

Lapham's Quarterly, *Death*, Fall 2013, Vol. VI, Number 4.

Levitin, Daniel J. *This is your brain on music*. Plume, 2006.

Lo, Bernard. *Resolving ethical dilemmas*. Lippincott Williams & Wilkins, 2013.

Lynch, Thomas. *Bodies in motion and at rest*. New York. Norton, 2000.

Meyer, Stephen C. *Return of the God Hypothesis*. Harper One, 2021.

Montross, Christine. *The Body of Work*. Penguin Press, 2000.

Nadler, Steven. *The best of all possible worlds*. Farrar, Straus & Garoux, 2008.

Nagel, Thomas. *What does it all mean*. Oxford University Press, 1989.

Nozick, Robert. *The examined life: Philosophical meditations*. New York: Simon & Schuster, 2006.

Nuland, Sherwin B. *How we die*. Knopf, 1994.

O'Connor, Maeve, Wolstenholme, GEW. *Ethics in Medical Progress with Special Reference to Transplantation.* Churchill, 1966.

Pellegrino, Ed, Thomasma, DC. *The virtues in medical practice.* Oxford University Press, 1993.

Pellegrino, Ed. *The trials of Job: a physician's meditation.* Linacre Quarterly, May 1989, pp. 76-80.

Rosenberg, Jay. *Thinking clearly about death.* Prentice-Hall, 1983.

Sadegh-Zadeh, Kazem. *Handbook of Analytic Philosophy of Medicine.* Springer Dordrecht, 2015.

Samtur, Stephen M. and Jackson, Martin A. *The Bronx 1935-1975.* Back in the Bronx, 1999.

Spiro, Howard M. *Facing Death.* Yale University Press, 1996.

Stone, John and Reynolds, Richard. *On Doctoring.* New York: Simon & Schuster, 1999.

ABOUT THE AUTHOR

Raised in a Bronx Italian-American home, Frank J. Brescia, MD, MA, attended Fordham University and Rutgers Medical School, later serving as a fellow in medical oncology at Memorial Hospital Sloan Kettering. His Vietnam War infantry service deeply influenced his perspective on death. Personal loss, including of his wife, Jane, following her battle with breast cancer, further shaped his understanding of love, grief, and the human condition. Holding a master's in philosophy from Fordham, he combines his medical expertise with philosophical insights, offering a unique viewpoint on life's profound challenges. This journey of discovery and reflection is evident in his thought-provoking writings.

ACKNOWLEDGEMENTS

I am grateful to a great number of people who provided me insight, feedback, and constructive criticism while writing this manuscript. My dear friends John Farrauto, and Dr. Russel Portenoy gave me initial encouragement- that this project was worth the effort. I wish to thank my cousin, Dr. Robert Brescia, for his multiple readings and comments. I am grateful to my lifetime critic Dr. Jerald Graff for pointing out all my mistakes and directing me to the right place. I am deeply humbled by my daughter Monica Brescia and owe her an enormous amount of thanks for always keeping me on track to use a better word, an improved phrase, and enhance my clarity of thought. I need to thank my mother in law Charlie McElroy who read the manuscript and gave me undo praise. My typist Mira Clavecilla -now a medical student- made the whole process so much easier for me. Christie always stopped to listen to my work in progress with patience, time, and praise. I thank my oncology nursing staff for pushing me and asking "When will this be finished?" I thank you Jane for everything.